Radionuclide Imaging Techniques

MEDICAL PHYSICS SERIES

P. N. T. WELLS. Physical Principles of Ultrasonic Diagnosis. 1969

D. W. HILL and A. M. DOLAN. Intensive Care Instrumentation (2nd edition). 1982

P. N. T. WELLS. Biomedical Ultrasonics. 1977

P. ROLFE. Non-invasive Physiological Measurements. Volume 1. 1979

P. ATKINSON and J. P. WOODCOCK. Doppler Ultrasound and its Use in Clinical Measurement. 1981

P. ROLFE. Non-invasive Physiological Measurements. Volume 2. 1983

A. R. WILLIAMS. Ultrasound: Biological Effects and Potential Hazards. 1983

G. LASZLO and M. F. SUDLOW (eds). Measurement of Clinical Respiratory Physiology. 1983

PETER F. SHARP, PHILIP P. DENDY, and W. IAN KEYES. Radionuclide Imaging Techniques. 1985

Contents

Chapter 5   Measurement of Imaging Device Performance

Chapter 6   Other Imaging Devices

Chapter 7   Image Display

Chapter 8   Data Analysis

Preface

Over the past 25 years, *in vivo* imaging of small quantities of radioactive materials for the purpose of diagnosis has developed into an important subject in its own right and has become the major area of nuclear medicine. The present state of the subject is the result of successful collaboration by many disciplines but notably by physicists and clinicians. Physicists have made important contributions in the past, and since the production of good-quality images will always depend on strict adherence to sound physical principles, the opportunity to contribute now and in the future provides a challenge to any physicist willing to study the problems. This book examines the current corpus of knowledge and prospects for the future from the physicist's viewpoint.

To review the subject in this way is timely because nuclear medicine is pausing after a period of rapid development. During the past 10 years, there have been dramatic improvements in the performance of imaging devices, and the introduction of dedicated data processing facilities has resulted in a rapid growth of dynamic investigations to alternative technologies. At the same time there has been some loss of the older static investigations to alternative technologies.

The current growth of nuclear medicine is primarily the extension of existing technology to more and more hospitals. In the future, some new diagnostic procedures will undoubtedly be introduced, particularly with the development of better radiopharmaceuticals, and even greater use of data processing techniques is anticipated.

In this book we examine three important aspects of radionuclide imaging. First, what is the nature of the image, and what are the physical principles behind its formation? Second, what factors determine the quality of the image, what factors limit the quality, and how should we establish physical criteria for assessing the quality? Finally, what is the value of the image? Is it providing useful clinical information, and how should we attempt to improve the image in order to improve the quality of that information?

The emphasis throughout is on those aspects that are most likely to interest, and it is hoped stimulate, physicists already working in nuclear medicine or those about to embark on a career in this area. We hope it may also be of interest to technologists and clinicians who are interested in the physical principles underlying the technique of radionuclide imaging.

Chapter 1

Introduction

The use of small quantities of radioactive material for diagnostic tests on patients has been practiced for more than 50 years. One of the earliest, if not the first such study, was reported by Blumgart and Yens (1927), who measured the arm-to-arm circulation time using a few millicuries (about 100 MBq) of radium-C. The beta emissions were detected with a Wilson cloud chamber.

Early progress was severely restricted by the limited choice of radio-nuclides (Hamilton, 1941), but by 1946 it was already clear that develop-ments which had taken place in connection with the use of atomic energy for military purposes during the Second World War would have a profound effect in medicine. Mitchell (1946) was able to list 36 artificially produced radionuclides which appeared to be of interest for biomedical investiga-tions. Production of selected radionuclides by means of a cyclotron was already being considered, and the importance of the short half-life nuclides, 11-carbon (11-C) (half-life 20.5 min), 13-nitrogen (13-N) (half-life 9.9 min), and 18-fluorine (18-F) (half-life 112 min), had been recog-nised. Medical applications under consideration at that time were uses as tracers and possibilities for therapy. Extension to *in vivo* imaging was to come later.

One important consequence of the advent of a wide range of artificially produced radionuclides was the much greater freedom of choice of both physical half-life and type of decay process. Depending upon the type of investigation envisaged, either a short physical half-life or a long physical half-life may be desirable. For example, if counting statistics and radiation dose to the patient are to be comparable, a short half-life will allow higher activities to be administered and imaging time can be reduced, whilst a long half-life may facilitate production, testing and distribution of a suitable radiopharmaceutical. With regard to the mode of decay, neither alpha nor negative beta particle emission is desirable, even if there is an associated gamma ray of suitable energy, because of the high radiation dose to the patient. Thus, it is necessary to consider alternative processes such as isomeric transitions (gamma ray decay or internal conversion) and isobaric transitions (positron decay or electron capture). For full details of these processes the reader should refer to a good text-book on nuclear physics (see, e.g., Burcham, 1973; Wagner, 1968).

Early pioneering work on *in vivo* imaging was generally carried out in centres where there was a cyclotron. Brain tumour detection was an early objective, and for this work positron-emitting nuclides were usually preferred to simple gamma emitters. At the end of the track of a positron, two 0.51-MeV gamma ray photons are emitted simultaneously in almost exactly opposite directions. If two opposed detectors are used, each may register an annihilation photon, and by using a coincidence circuit it can be arranged that only simultaneous pulses are recorded. Randomly directed radiation resulting from scatter and background can be eliminated. The degree of localisation and, hence, image definition that could be obtained in this way was better than by single-channel gamma ray counting with a simple conical collimator using 131-iodine (131-I), the gamma emitter then most generally available. Effective detection of brain tumours was achieved by Sweet *et al.* (1959) using 74-arsenic (74-As) and 64-copper (64-Cu) and by Mallard *et al.* (1961) using 72-arsenic (72-As).

The much greater yields of radionuclides obtainable with a reactor and the production of pure gamma emitters with much better physical properties were significant factors in determining subsequent developments. 99m-Technetium (99m-Tc), which has a 6-h half-life and emits almost monoenergetic gamma rays at 140 keV, is now the nuclide of choice for over 90% of *in vivo* imaging investigations (see Table 1.1). Reasons for this will be discussed in detail in Chapter 2. Nevertheless, minicyclotrons capable of producing small quantities of radionuclides for diagnostic studies are now available and there is considerable renewed interest in biologically important short half-life positron emitters such as 11-C and 13-N (Wagner, 1981).

Now that a wide variety of radionuclides is available, attention has focussed on the preparation of radiopharmaceuticals which show high selectivity in the organ of interest. Poor selectivity results in unwanted radioactivity above and below the region of interest with rapid deteriora-

TABLE 1.1. Ten of the most frequently performed imaging investigations.

Examination	Radionuclide	Static/dynamic	Principal application
Bone	99m-Tc	S	Secondary spread of malignancy
Liver	99m-Tc	S	Secondary spread of malignancy; cirrhotic changes
Brain	99m-Tc	S/D	Occult metastases; brain damage; vascular problems
Lung (perfusion)	99m-Tc	S	Pulmonary embolism
Lung (ventilation)	133-Xe/99m-Tc	D	Pulmonary emphysema
Kidneys	123-I/99m-Tc	D	Renal function
Hepato-biliary system	99m-Tc	D	Patency of the biliary tree; liver function
Thyroid	123-I/99m-Tc	S	Thyroid function
Heart (perfusion)	201-Tl	S	Cardiac infarction and ischaemia
Heart (blood pool)	99m-Tc	D	Cardiac wall motion

tion in the signal to noise ratio. This topic will also be considered in detail in Chapter 2.

The earliest attempts to develop *in vivo* imaging involved mapping the distribution of radioactivity using hand-held Geiger counters. For example, Ansell and Rotblat (1948) published a point-by-point determination of 131-I distribution obtained in this way for an intrathoracic goitre. In the same year, Moore (1948) reported an early attempt to diagnose and localise brain tumours after administration of 131-I diiodofluorescein using a hand-held Geiger counter at different positions on the skull. However, the origins of *in vivo* imaging as we know it today can be traced back to the development of suitable scintillation detectors. The technique of scintillation counting had been one of Rutherford's most powerful weapons for the study of atomic nuclei (Rutherford *et al.*, 1930) but at that time it was thought that only alpha particles, not beta particles or gamma rays, could cause this effect. Subsequently, with the development of better scintillants, it was found that scintillations from beta and gamma rays could be detected readily, especially if the crystal was cooled to reduce noise. For an excellent account of the medical applications of scintillation counting at that time, the reader is referred to Mayneord and Belcher (1950).

Cassen *et al.* (1951) reported the first attempt to obtain a direct image of a body organ by way of emitted radiation. A single rod of calcium tungstate was used to record the gamma rays, and the thyroid images obtained after administration of 131-I were surprisingly good, although history does not actually record the dose given to patients. At a symposium arranged by the Institute of Electrical Engineers in 1950, two papers (Sharpe and Taylor, 1951; Owen and Sayle, 1951) discussed the use of thallium-activated sodium iodide crystals [NaI(Tl)] in scintillation detectors, and within a couple of years reports were appearing of the use of this scintillant, or its close analogue thallium-activated potassium iodide, for *in vivo* work (Anger, 1952; Belcher *et al.*, 1952). The properties of NaI(Tl) that make it particularly suitable for *in vivo* imaging will be discussed in Chapter 2. It is of interest to note that some 30 years later this is still the scintillant of choice in all commercial imaging devices.

From this early work, quite separate types of specialised study developed. The most important is static imaging whereby high-resolution techniques are used to give the best possible image of the organ of interest. For this purpose two basically different designs of imaging device were developed, the rectilinear scanner and the gamma camera. The rectilinear scanner is older and simpler in concept. It normally consists of two detectors, arranged one above and one below the patient. The detectors are coupled to the same mechanical movement, which, by means of an $x-y$ raster motion, is able to scan systematically over a preselected area. Each detector consists of an NaI(Tl) crystal coupled to a single photomultiplier tube (PMT). Positional data is obtained simply by correlating the recorded count rate with the spatial position of the detectors at that time. Both the scan speed and the raster line spacing can be adjusted by the operator, depending upon the area of the body that is to be scanned and the amount of activity it contains. As the gamma rays recorded at a particular instant are assumed to originate only from that part of the patient directly below the detector, it is necessary to restrict the field of view. This is done by placing in front of each detector a collimator consisting of a block of high density material, usually lead, with an array of tapered holes running through it. These holes are arranged so that they focus at a point some distance in front of the collimator. Gamma rays emitted from the small volume of tissue around the focal point will have the highest probability of being detected; the smaller this "in focus" volume, the sharper the resulting images. Good collimator design is essential for high quality images and will be considered in Chapter 3.

The suggestion that a gamma-ray camera could image *in vivo* distributions of radioactivity (Anger, 1957, 1958) was eventually to revolutionize the subject. The camera is a stationary device and depends for its operation on a different imaging principle from the scanner. In particular it allows a large surface area of scintillation crystal to be exposed to gamma rays, and in modern cameras the crystal can be up to 60 cm in diameter.

This is important because the imaging process is severely photon limited by restrictions on the amount of radioactive material that can be administered to the patient.

To form an image, the gamma rays must first be collimated. Gamma camera collimators usually consist of an array of parallel holes separated by lead septa, so that only those gamma rays travelling perpendicular to the crystal face are detected. A relationship now exists between the position of the scintillation and the origin of the gamma ray. The image formed on the crystal consists of a series of brief scintillations and in this form is unsuitable for viewing or recording. Therefore, the spatial position and energy associated with each scintillation is measured electronically by an array of PMTs behind the crystal. In modern cameras there may be between 37 and 91 PMTs. After electronic manipulation, including pulse height analysis, the signals are used to produce a visible flash of light on a cathode ray tube display. These flashes can then be integrated on photographic film to form a permanent image. The gamma camera has now virtually replaced the rectilinear scanner for imaging, and full details of its design will be given in Chapter 3.

The first studies to be performed were static images showing the distribution of radiopharmaceutical once it had been concentrated in the structure of interest. However, the potential for performing dynamic studies, in which changes in distribution of the radiopharmaceutical are monitored throughout the investigation, was recognised at an early stage (see, e.g., Potchen *et al.*, 1969). Initially such studies were restricted to measuring the variation in count rate at certain pre-selected areas of the body using simple probe detectors. This approach produced much useful information, particularly in renal investigations, but the lack of an imaging capability had obvious disadvantages.

Two developments were essential before dynamic imaging could be contemplated as a routine study. The first development was an imaging device with a reasonably large field of view that was sufficiently sensitive to give statistically meaningful counts for short time frames. The gamma camera satisfies these requirements, but for dynamic imaging a collimator design which increases sensitivity at the expense of some loss of resolution is frequently chosen. The second development was the availability of reasonably priced data handling hardware and software powerful enough to process the very large amount of data being collected. The latter development has only occurred during the past 10 years and dynamic radionuclide imaging as a readily available routine investigation in most smaller hospitals only dates from the late 1970s.

The third and rather more specialised technique that will be considered briefly in Chapter 3 in ultrahigh-sensitivity low-resolution whole-body imaging. This is an imaging version of the whole-body counter in which extremely high sensitivity is required so that very small quantities of radioactive material such as 40-potassium (40-K), which occurs naturally in the body, or ingested radioactivity, e.g., 125-I from occupational exposure, may be detected. Image quality is correspondingly poor, but under favourable conditions the distribution of radioactivity can be localised approximately.

Unwanted signals arising from activity in planes above and below the region of interest have already been mentioned. This is a problem that is not confined to radionuclide imaging, and the term tomography has been applied to techniques aimed at visualising one layer or section of the body with little or no interference from adjacent layers. Two techniques have evolved, and for convenience these are termed "longitudinal" and "transverse" tomography. In longitudinal tomography, details in one chosen plane are kept in focus whilst attempts are made to blur detail from other planes. In transverse tomography, information is collected from a single plane by viewing it from several different directions, and an image is reconstructed from this information using mathematical techniques implemented by digital computer. It is interesting to record that transverse tomography was used in radionuclide imaging (Kuhl and Edwards, 1963) a decade before the introduction of the very successful X-ray transmission-scanner (Hounsfield, 1973). However, transverse radionuclide emission imaging did not involve any fundamental change in the equipment whereas the X-ray transmission method involved a very fundamental change of two vital pieces of equipment, the detector and the method of display. The unique section view produced led to a fundamental increase in the accuracy of X-ray measurement in diagnostic radiology. Although tomographic techniques have not made as big an impact on nuclear medicine as on radiology, they have made an important contribution and will be considered in some detail in Chapter 4.

An important goal has been to establish appropriate parameters for assessing imaging device performance. There is now general agreement that, from a physical viewpoint, the most relevant are sensitivity, spatial and temporal resolution, spatial linearity, uniformity and energy resolution. However, evaluation cannot be made in purely physical terms without due consideration of the practical problems associated with clinical investigations. These factors will all be considered in Chapter 5.

The major deficiencies of current imaging devices are relatively poor spatial resolution, which is closely related to poor energy resolution, and poor performance at high count rates. While the NaI(Tl) crystal remains the basic detecting device, opportunities for significant improvement are limited since the constraints are imposed primarily by the physical principles involved in the gamma ray detection process. One possibility is to increase the area of NaI(Tl) crystal surrounding the patient, thereby trapping a greater percentage of gamma rays. Sensitivity is thus increased and, by suitable collimator design, some of this improved sensitivity can be traded off for improved resolution. In another approach, count-rate performance has been improved by replacing the single large crystal by an array of small crystals. Positional information is obtained simply by identifying the crystal in which the photo-electric event occurred, and this is a much faster process. Poor energy resolution results from the relatively small number of visible light photons released by each gamma ray. Recently some prototypes have replaced the scintillation crystals with semiconductor detectors which give a high yield of electron/holes for each gamma-ray conversion. Finally, the use of a collimator is a severe limitation because it greatly reduces sensitivity, and several alternatives have been suggested. For example, coded apertures, in particular Fresnel zone plates, offer one possibility, using a standard scintillation detector or even X-ray film for data recording. An alternative approach has been to determine the point of origin of the gamma ray by measuring the trajectory and energy loss of Compton scattered gamma rays, a so-called Compton-effect camera. Collimators can also be dispensed with by using coincidence systems for positron detection, but this approach has the disadvantage of requiring an on-site cyclotron to produce most of the biologically important radionuclides. These and other potential developments will be discussed in Chapter 6.

So far this introduction has been concerned with data collection. However, it is important to appreciate that, although the performance of an imaging device can be measured by comparing the count density pattern it produces with the actual distribution of radiopharmaceutical, effectiveness in the clinical environment depends also upon how well the data are presented to the clinician. Therefore, other important aspects of the full diagnostic procedure are image display, analysis and interpretation. A variety of displays is possible with all imaging devices. The oldest, used in conjunction with a scanner, is the dot density display where a mark is made by a mechanical tapper hitting an inked ribbon each time a gamma ray is detected. By moving the tapper unit in synchronism with the detector, a monochrome or grey scale intensity pattern is produced. A wide variety of displays is now used to show data in colour as well as monochrome. Furthermore, since data handling by computer-interfaced systems is now employed widely, there is a general trend away from analogue towards digital displays. The methods that are currently favoured will

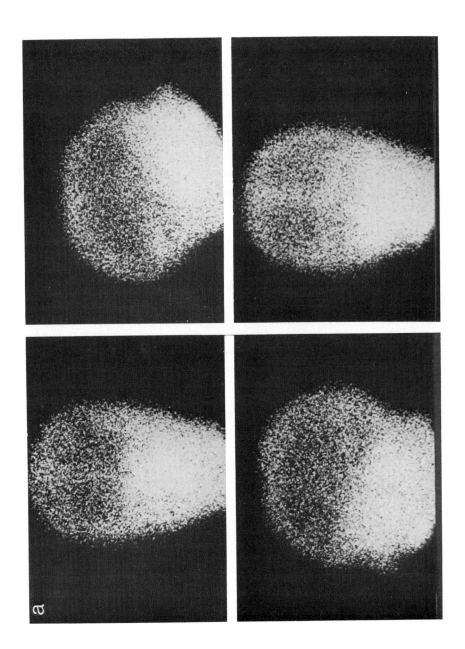

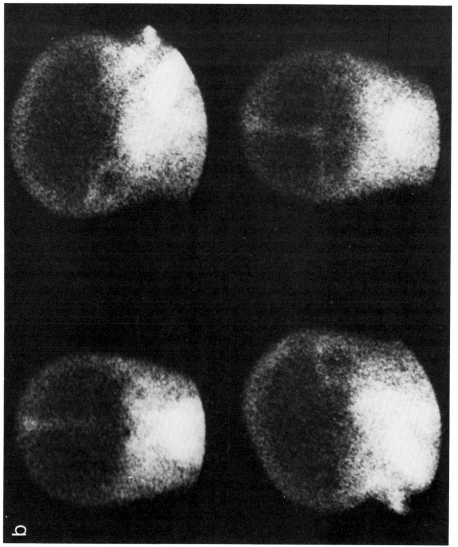

Fig. 1.1. Brain scan performed with a gamma camera: (a) in 1968 and (b) in 1984. (Courtesy of Dr. F. W. Smith, Aberdeen Royal Infirmary.)

be presented in Chapter 7, and some important problems associated with data analysis, including data reduction, image filtering and quantitation of radiopharmaceutical uptake, will be discussed in Chapter 8.

The final topic will be evaluation of clinical images. It is perhaps surprising that this aspect of *in vivo* imaging has been neglected for so long and that medical physicists in particular are only now beginning to respond to the fact that the design of high quality imaging equipment is only a means to an end, not an end in itself. Few attempts have been made to design clinical trials that will compare the ultimate accuracy of different diagnostic approaches, or even minor variations in basically the same approach, for example, in the method of data display. Such trials are not easy to design and occasionally may prove impossible. However, new and ever more expensive technologies are continually being developed so the need for critical evaluation becomes increasingly important. The contribution of an expensive new technique must be evaluated not only in terms of its diagnostic accuracy but also in terms of its influence on patient management. Careful trials are required to verify that the added information, not readily acquired by traditional methods, warrants the extra cost involved. This book would not be complete without some consideration of these problems.

The concluding chapter will summarise the key features of the current state of the art and speculate on future developments. Figure 1.1 illustrates dramatically the progress that has been made in the last twenty years. This rate of progress cannot be maintained, but we hope to identify some areas in which *in vivo* radionuclide imaging has unrealised potential.

References

Anger, H. O. (1952). Use of gamma ray pinhole camera for *in vivo* studies. *Nature* (*London*) **1170**, 200–201.

Anger, H. O. (1957). A new instrument for mapping gamma ray emitters. *Biol. Med. Q. Rep. UCRL* **UCRL-3653**, 38.

Anger, H. O. (1958). Scintillation camera. *Rev. Sci. Instrum.* **29**, 27–33.

Ansell G. and Rotblat, J. (1948). Radioactive iodine as a diagnostic aid for intrathoracic goitre. *Br. J. Radiol.* **21**, 552–558.

Belcher, E. H., Evans, H. S. and de Winter, J. G. (1952). Use of radioactive diiodofluorescein for the attempted localisation of brain tumours. *Br. Med. Bull.* **8**, 172–180.

Blumgart, H. L. and Yens, O. C. (1927). Studies on the velocity of blood flow. 1. The method utilised. *J. Clin. Invest.* **4**, 1–13.

Burcham, W. E. (1973). "Nuclear Physics—An Introduction", 2nd Ed. Longmans, London.

Cassen, B., Curtis, L., Reid, C. and Libby, R. (1951). 131-I use in medical studies. *Nucleonics* **9**, 46–50.

Hamilton, J. G. (1941). The application of radioactive tracers to medicine and biology. *J. Appl. Phys.* **12**, 440–460.

Hounsfield, G. N. (1973). Computerised transvere axial scanning (tomography). Pt. 1. Description of system. *Br. J. Radiol.* **46**, 1016–1022.

Kuhl, D. E. and Edwards, R. Q. (1963). Image separation radioisotope scanning. *Radiology* **80**, 653–661.

Mallard, J. R., Fowler, J. F. and Sutton, M. (1961). Brain tumour detection using radioactive arsenic. *Br. J. Radiol.* **34**, 562–568.

Mayneord, W. V. and Belcher, E. H. (1950). Scintillation counting and its medical application. *In* "Some Applications of Nuclear Physics to Medicine". *Br. J. Radiol.*, *Suppl.* 2, 251–290.

Mitchell, J. S. (1946). Applications of recent advances in nuclear physics to medicine. *Br. J. Radiol.* **19**, 481–487.

Moore, G. E. (1948). Use of radioactive diiodofluorescein in the diagnosis and localisation of brain tumours. *Science (Washington, D.C.)* **107**, 569–571.

Owen, R. B. and Sayle, E. A. (1951). Scintillation counting equipment. *Proc. Inst. Electr. Eng.* **98**, Part II, 245–251.

Potchen, E. J., Bentley, R. E., Gerth, W., Hill, R. L. and Davis, D. O. (1969). A means for the scintigraphic imaging of regional brain dynamics. *In* "Medical Radioisotope Scintigraphy", Vol. 2, pp. 557–583. IAEA, Vienna.

Rutherford, E, Chadwick, J. and Ellis, C. D. (1930). "Radiations from Radioactive Substances". Cambridge University Press, London.

Sharpe, J. and Taylor, D. (1951). Nuclear particle and radiation detectors. Part 2. Counters and counting system. *Proc. Inst. Electr. Eng.* **98**, Part II, 209–230.

Sweet, W. H., Meadley, J., Brownell, G. L. and Aronow, S. (1959). Coincidence scanning with positron emitting arsenic or copper in the diagnosis of focal intracranial disease. *In* "Medical Radioisotope Scanning", pp. 163–183. IAEA, Vienna.

Wagner, H. N., Jr. (1968). "Principles of Nuclear Medicine". W. B. Saunders, Philadelphia, Pennsylvania.

Wagner, H. N., Jr. (1981). New perspectives in nuclear imaging. *In* "Medical Radionuclide Imaging 1980", Vol. 1, pp. 3–26. IAEA, Vienna.

Chapter 2

The Imaging Problem

There are many factors that contribute to the formation of a good radionuclide image and its correct interpretation. The most fundamental of these will be considered in this chapter. In the first part of this chapter a simple mathematical model will be used to investigate how various physical factors, such as the energy of the photons, influence image quality. In the second part of the chapter an equally fundamental problem, that of the correct choice of radiopharmaceutical, will be considered with particular emphasis on the properties required of an ideal radionuclide and how it can be complexed with various pharmaceuticals to give a highly selective uptake in the organ of interest.

2.1 The physical aspect

Our aim is to form an image of a distribution of radionuclide within a patient, using the emitted radiation detectable at the surface of the patient. The emitted radiation is invariably X or gamma radiation, arising either directly from nuclear disintegration or indirectly via positron emission. In practice very little of this radiation can be used to form an image. Photon density in radionuclide imaging is of the order of 10^2 cm^{-2} compared with about 10^7 cm^{-2} in radiography and 10^{12} cm^{-2} in conventional photography. One important consequence is that the statistical fluctuations in photon density inherent in radioactive decay will affect image quality. This results in variations in photon density even when the distribution of radionuclide is uniform. Consequently, only those changes in the radiopharmaceutical distribution which are greater than statistical noise will be detectable.

Not only are radionuclide images noisy, but they can only be produced with relatively poor spatial resolution, about 1 cm. Thus, in comparison with most other types of images, radionuclide images are of very poor quality.

2.1.1 The detection problem

A simple mathematical model can be developed to aid our understanding of the general problem. The model provides a quantitative appreciation of the magnitude of various effects and the inter-relationships of the many physical parameters involved. Figure 2.1 illustrates the simplest imaging task, that of identifying the presence of a region of different radioactivity concentration within a constant background. The following assumptions are made:

(i) there is a background region of total depth L, containing a radionuclide concentration (activity per unit volume) C_b, and a target consisting of a spherical region of diameter d, at depth t, with a different concentration C_t,

(ii) the radionuclide emits gamma rays with attenuation coefficient μ in the medium which is assumed to be unit density tissue,

(iii) there is pure exponential attenuation of gamma rays in the medium,

(iv) the detector accepts all gamma rays incident normal to its surface with equal efficiency

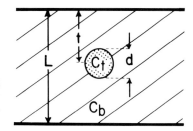

FIG. 2.1. Model of the simplest imaging problem–identifying a region of radioactivity concentration C_t within a constant background C_b.

(v)   the signal to noise ratio (where the noise is simply the statistical fluctuation of the count rate over the background and the signal is the change in count rate directly over the target) is an adequate measure of detectability of the target.

The count rate in the detector is thus a measure of the flux of gamma rays emitted perpendicular to its surface. These conditions are, of course, rarely achieved in practice (although they represent a reasonable approximation to the response of a gamma camera equipped with a parallel-hole collimator or a rectilinear scanner with a long-focus collimator).

Consider a narrow cylinder of cross-sectional area dA in the background region. The number of gamma rays per unit time dN at the surface will be given by

$$dN \propto \int_0^L C_b \, dA \, \exp(-\mu z) \, dz \qquad (2.1)$$

where dz is the thickness of an element of the cylinder at depth z measured from the surface, and $C_b \, dA \, dz$ is the activity in this element. Thus, for the flux over the background region we may write

$$\frac{dN}{dA} \propto C_b \int_0^L \exp(-\mu z) \, dz = \frac{C_b[1 - \exp(-\mu L)]}{\mu} \qquad (2.2)$$

and since the count rate in the detector will be proportional to this value, we have for the "background count rate per unit area of detector", R_b,

$$R_b = (kC_b)[1 - \exp(-\mu L)]/\mu \qquad (2.3)$$

The constant of proportionality k represents the sensitivity of the detector. At this stage all that sensitivity implies is the ability of the detector to convert gamma ray flux to count rate per unit area. A more specific definition of sensitivity follows later.

The change in count rate per unit area due to the target, i.e., the signal R_s, is likewise given by

$$R_s = k(C_t - C_b) \int_{t-d/2}^{t+d/2} \exp(-\mu z) \, dz$$
$$= k(C_t - C_b)\{\exp[-\mu(t - d/2)] - \exp[-\mu(t + d/2)]\}/\mu \quad (2.4)$$

The variation of count rate from point to point over the detector combined with the integration time (or exposure time) T leads to an image in which the count density pattern represents the spatial distribution of the activity integrated over depth L, the conventional radionuclide image.

The target will be detectable provided a significantly different count density is observed over the target area compared to the background area. To obtain actual numbers of counts we must now specify an area of the detector surface and look at counts within this area when it is positioned first over the background and then directly over the target. For simplicity, assume this area Δ to be small in comparison to the target. Now since the noise is described by Poisson statistics, it will be proportional to the square root of the background counts $\sqrt{TR_b\Delta}$. The signal will be proportional to $TR_s\Delta$ so we have, using Eqs. (2.3) and (2.4), an expression for the signal to noise ratio (SNR)

$$\text{SNR} = TR_s\Delta/\sqrt{TR_b\Delta} \tag{2.5}$$

$$= \frac{k^{1/2}T^{1/2}\,\Delta^{1/2}(C_t - C_b)\{\exp[-\mu(t - d/2)] - \exp[-\mu(t + d/2)]\}}{C_b^{1/2}[1 - \exp(-\mu L)]^{1/2}}$$

We can thus investigate how the detectability of the target will depend on the particular imaging problem.

The variables C_b and C_t are essentially biochemical, depending on the uptake of radionuclide in the target and surroundings. The remaining terms are purely physical, depending on the sensitivity of the detector, the time spent collecting counts, the area Δ, the attenuation of gamma rays in the medium and the geometry of the problem. The area Δ cannot be increased indefinitely to improve the SNR, since the expression for the signal [Eq. (2.4)] only applies to the centre of the target.

The form of Eq. (2.5) tells us much about radionuclide imaging requirements. In order to double the SNR, we need a fourfold increase in sensitivity or time. These are characteristic features of radionuclide counting in general. Also to visualise tumours we need substances which give a large value of $(C_t - C_b)/C_b^{1/2}$, i.e., good differential concentration between tumour and its surroundings and low background concentration. Tumour-specific compounds have been sought for many years. Ideally, if C_b tends to zero then SNR becomes infinite, so any uptake at all in the tumour would be detectable and radionuclide imaging would provide a screening test with 100% accuracy. However, detection of very low levels of radioactivity would always be limited by radiation from the environment, and in practice with compounds developed to date, C_b is substantially non-zero. It is the statistical uncertainty in the measurement of C_b which gives rise to the noise level.

The differential concentration is more often expressed as a concentration ratio C_t/C_b. Rearranging the terms in Eq. (2.5) we have

$$\text{SNR} \propto C_b^{1/2}(C_t/C_b - 1) \tag{2.6}$$

Concentration ratios between 0 and 1 indicate that the target concentration is less than the background. Note that a "void" ($C_t = 0$) gives the same value of SNR (but with opposite sign) as a target with concentration ratio of 2. Note also that for a given concentration ratio C_t/C_b, SNR will be proportional to $C_b^{1/2}$; in other words to double the SNR requires four times the amount of activity, again characteristic of radionuclide counting in general.

We can use this simple model to show how the physical variables affect detectability. Equation (2.5) should tell us which value of μ, and hence energy of gamma ray, produces the best detectability. Figure 2.2 illustrates the variation of SNR with μ for various geometries. Generally the best

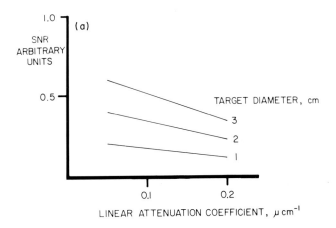

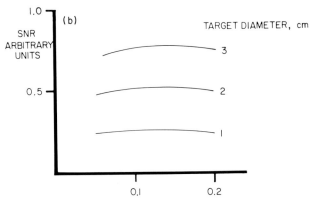

Fig. 2.2. Variation of signal to noise ratio with μ for different geometries: (a) targets 7 cm deep in total depth 20 cm and (b) targets 3 cm deep in total depth 20 cm.

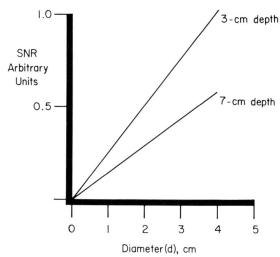

FIG. 2.3. Variation of signal to noise ratio with diameter of target when $\mu = 0.14 \text{ cm}^{-1}$ and $L = 20 \text{ cm}$.

SNR is obtained with small values of μ (higher energy of gamma ray), but note that superficial targets in fairly deep backgrounds are best detected with specific values of μ. Thus, for example with a 2-cm diameter target, 3 cm deep in a background 20 cm thick, a broad peak is observed with optimum μ equal to 0.14 cm^{-1} equivalent to the attenuation of 140-keV gamma rays in water. In a more comprehensive investigation of detectability as a function of photon energy, collimator design must also be taken into account (Chapter 3). Figures 2.3 and 2.4 show that for fixed concentration, SNR increases as the target diameter increases and decreases as the depth increases.

As a final application of this simple model, we can investigate how the concentration ratio required for a given level of detectability varies with diameter of target (Fig. 2.5). The increase of SNR for increasing diameter of target in Fig. 2.3 can be reduced by decreasing the concentration ratio such that a fixed SNR is achieved. We then find that a steep increase in concentration ratio is required to maintain SNR as the diameter of the target shrinks. However, detectability of very small targets is possible given a sufficiently high concentration ratio.

Whilst the preceding is instructive in providing inter-relationships between the main variables, the validity of the conclusions depends on the initial assumptions. Two of these must be examined very critically. First, practical detectors do not accept all gamma rays incident normally with equal efficiency. Secondly, the clinical problem is much more complex than that depicted in Fig. 2.1, since the medium is neither homogeneous nor

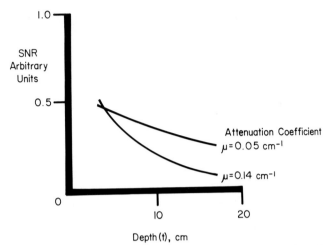

FIG. 2.4. Variation of signal to noise ratio with depth of target when $d = 2$ cm and $L = 20$ cm.

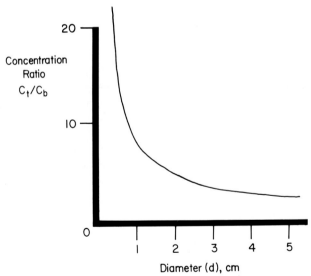

FIG. 2.5. Illustration of how the concentration ratio required for a given arbitrary level of detectability varies with target diameter, all other parameters being equal.

likely to provide a background of uniform concentration in which to estimate the presence of a likely target. Under clinical conditions, anatomical uncertainties provide additional noise so that even higher signals will be required.

However, the preceding idealised considerations can provide a lower limit on which to estimate the detectability of targets. It is worth emphasizing that detectability in radionuclide imaging is very much a signal to noise ratio problem and that decreasing noise is as important as increasing the signal. If an increase in the signal, e.g., by a new innovation or technique, is accompanied by a substantial increase in noise, there may well be no net gain in terms of lesion detectability and, hence, no improvement in imaging capability.

2.1.2 The resolution problem

To improve our understanding further we must now consider the detector itself and accept that the problem is not simply to detect the presence of a region of different radioactivity concentration but also to identify the target and to delineate its structure if possible. We must refine our mathematical model to take account of the field of view at each point over the detector surface. The finite size of this field of view gives rise to the spatial resolution of the system and is also fundamental in determining the real sensitivity of practical detectors.

In Eq. (2.2) we considered the gamma ray flux dN/dA as producing a count rate proportional to this value at an individual point on the detector surface. We assumed that the detector accepted all gamma rays incident normal to its surface. To allow for the detection of non-normal incident gamma rays, which will occur in all practical collimation systems, we can associate a solid angle W with each point on the detector surface (Fig. 2.6). The sensitivity of the system can now be improved by increasing W, the penalty being a decrease in resolving ability. Since W is small we can still assume proportionality between counting rate per unit area and the gamma ray flux dN/dA, and we can assume direct proportionality between W and sensitivity [i.e., k of Eq. (2.3) is now the sensitivity per unit solid angle]. Thus, in the very simplest terms, we can investigate how systems with different resolution would perform the same imaging task. To avoid complications of integrating in three dimensions we will limit the objects to a single plane and again consider a background region of concentration C_b per unit area and a target area with concentration C_t. By following the same arguments as before we can derive an expression for the SNR. Two separate cases can be identified:

(i)   the target is larger than acceptance cone ($r_t > r$); therefore, background counts $\propto k(\pi r^2)TC_b$ and signal counts $\propto k(\pi r^2)T(C_t - C_b)$ so,

$$\text{SNR} = k^{1/2}T^{1/2}\,(C_t - C_b)\pi^{1/2}r/C_b^{1/2} \qquad (2.7)$$

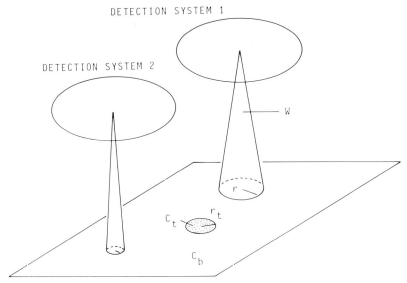

FIG. 2.6. Model for investigating how systems with different resolution would perform the same imaging task. The sensitivity of the detection system is proportional to the solid angle W, which subtends a circle of radius r (the resolution radius) at the object plane.

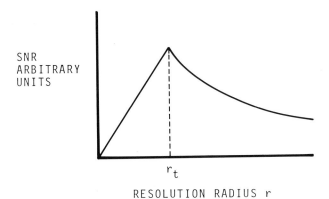

FIG. 2.7. Variation of signal to noise ratio with r, the resolution radius, for the detection of a circular target of radius r_t.

(ii) the target is smaller than acceptance cone $(r_t < r)$; therefore, background counts $\propto k(\pi r^2) T C_b$ and signal counts $\propto k(\pi r_t^2) T (C_t - C_b)$ so,

$$\text{SNR} = k^{1/2} T^{1/2} (C_t - C_b) \pi^{1/2} r_t^1 / C_b^{1/2} r \qquad (2.8)$$

Figure 2.7 combines these results and indicates the existence of an optimum resolution, matched to the task in hand. Practical systems do not have such well-defined acceptance cones, but meticulous theoretical and experimental work can still determine the optimum detector resolution for specific tasks (Tsui *et al.*, 1983). The resolution and sensitivity of an imaging system are largely determined by this "field of view" of each point on the detector surface. The signal to noise ratio is maximised when the field of view is matched to the diameter of the target. If some sort of target recognition is desired, then it is worthwhile to sacrifice some sensitivity for superior resolution.

Since tumours which cause symptoms in patients are usually over 1 cm in diameter, systems with this resolution evolved rapidly and proved useful. However, even better resolution, down to 5 mm in some circumstances, can now be achieved. While tumours of under 1 cm are rarely detected, this high resolution may be of value for imaging normal anatomical structure, i.e., for reducing anatomical noise.

2.1.3 Practical detectors

All we have required of our detector so far is the ability to convert gamma ray flux to count rate per unit area. To perform this function efficiently the detector must absorb a high proportion of the incident radiation and convert this energy rapidly into suitable electronic signals. If the energy of the incident radiation can be inferred from the electronic signals then energy analysis can be applied in order to discriminate against photons scattered within the patient. These secondary photons would be imaged as originating from the site of the Compton interaction. This degrades the information, since the object of the imaging procedure is to localise the site of the gamma emitting radionuclide itself.

At the present time thallium-activated sodium iodide NaI(Tl) scintillation crystals are used in all commercial imaging devices. The high density and high atomic number increase the probability that an incident gamma ray will be absorbed in the crystal. The high atomic number (53 for iodine) favours the photoelectric interaction. Thus, a signal is generated which represents the full energy of the gamma ray. Pulse height analysis can then be used to select photopeak events and reject scattered photons.

The presence of thallium in the crystal gives a conversion efficiency, i.e., the ratio of light output to incident photon energy, of about 10% for a 140-keV gamma ray. This is equivalent to converting the gamma ray into about 4200 light photons. The decay time of this light flash has a half-life of only 0.2 μsec. Thus the crystal is capable of handling the highest count rates encountered in clinical imaging without problems caused by scintillations overlapping each other.

The photomultiplier tube (PMT) is optically coupled to the scintillation crystal and converts the light output from the crystal to an electronic pulse. Of the light photons produced, only about 25% will actually be converted into electrons at the photocathode of the PMT. Statistical fluctuations in the number of electrons produced will be high thereby resulting in variations in the height of the pulse coming from the PMT. This limits the scintillation detector's energy resolution, i.e., the accuracy with which the energy of a gamma ray can be measured. As a result it is difficult to use pulse height analysis to exclude scattered gamma rays from the image.

Semi-conductor detectors constructed from silicon or germanium have been tried experimentally. Compared to NaI(Tl) crystals they have inherently superior energy resolution. This is a result of the direct transformation of photon energy into electrically charged carriers; typically a 140-keV gamma ray will produce about 50,000 electron/hole pairs.

Multiwire proportional chambers have also been tried experimentally. The low absorption of incident photons again leads to very low sensitivity in comparison to NaI(Tl). With high-pressure gas filling and converter foils it may be possible to make more practical use of these devices particularly as large area detectors. However, at present the sodium iodide scintillation crystal has retained its role as the most suitable detector for imaging devices.

2.1.4 Practical collimation

In practice, the geometrical approach used in Fig. 2.6 will be insufficient to study real imaging systems. Gamma rays cannot be focussed by any known means, so the sophistication of the optical lens is sadly missing in gamma ray imaging devices and the image must be formed by relatively crude collimation, which excludes from the detector of all gamma rays except those travelling in a preferred direction. In the rectilinear scanner, where the detector acts as a simple gamma-ray counter, the focussed collimator is designed to accept a large proportion of those gamma rays emitted from the volume of tissue around the focal point. In contrast, the purpose of the collimator on the gamma camera is to form an actual image in the detector crystal. The multiple parallel channels of the parallel-hole collimator, for example, will give a unique relationship between the location of the scintillation in the detector crystal and the line of origin of the gamma ray in the patient.

In both cases the size of the collimator hole, together with some inevitable penetration of the lead septa between holes, will result in gamma rays other than those travelling parallel to the axes of the holes reaching the detector. This will degrade image sharpness, the acceptance cone no longer having a well-defined edge. Further deterioration in sharpness is caused by Compton scatter of primary photons in the patient, the collimator and the detector crystal.

Resolution and sensitivity of an imaging device can be measured from the image it produces of a distribution of radiopharmaceutical approximating a delta function, the "impulse response". In Fig. 2.6, for example, the impulse response would be a step function (an all or nothing response) with the width of the step function proportional to the distance from the detector. As the point source moves over the plane, it is either seen or unseen depending on whether it is inside or outside the field of view. The impulse response is more normally termed the "point spread function" PSF(x, y, z). Choosing the detector as the plane $z = 0$, then at any distance z we have the point sensitivity response in that plane PSF(x, y), which is usually a radially symmetric function. In practice the Gaussian function is often a close approximation, and we will use this analytical form to develop the mathematical model (Fig. 2.8)

$$\text{PSF}(x,y) = P_0 \exp[-a^2(x^2 + y^2)] \tag{2.9}$$

The units of PSF are usually counts per second per unit area per unit activity. The "resolution index" R is defined as the full width at half-maximum response (FWHM), and hence for the Gaussian model

$$R^2 = 2.77/a^2 \tag{2.10}$$

The peak value P_0 and the resolution index R will both be functions of z.

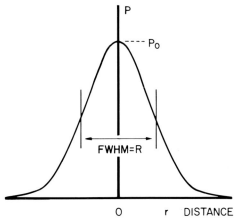

FIG 2.8. The idealised Gaussian point spread function $P = P_0 \exp(-a^2 r^2)$, where $r^2 = x^2 + y^2$ and $a^2 = 2.77/R^2$.

The integral of Eq. (2.9) in the y direction yields the "line spread function" (LSF), the response to a line source of radioactivity lying parallel to the y axis:

$$\text{LSF}(x) = \int_{-\infty}^{\infty} P_0(x,y)\,dy$$

$$= P_0 \exp(-a^2 x^2) \int_{-\infty}^{\infty} \exp(-a^2 y^2)\,dy$$

$$= P_0 \exp(-a^2 x^2)\pi^{1/2}/a \tag{2.11}$$

The usual units of LSF are counts per second per unit area per unit activity per unit length. The form of LSF (x) is thus seen to be identical to the form of PSF(x,y), with the same resolution index; and this result is usually found with practical collimators. Experimentally, a line source is easier to fabricate and handle; thus, the resolution index is conveniently measured using a line source.

The integral of Eq. (2.11) yields the plane source sensitivity, the response to an infinite plane of radioactivity

$$S_A = \int_{-\infty}^{\infty} \text{LSF}(x)\,dx = \frac{\pi P_0}{a^2} = \frac{\pi R^2 P_0}{2.77} \tag{2.12}$$

The units of S_A are then counts per second per unit activity. The plane sensitivity is of fundamental importance, since under ideal conditions it is independent of the distance between source and detector. The independence of plane sensitivity and distance can be appreciated from Fig. 2.6. The area of the plane source covered by the field of view increases in proportion to z^2 while the sensitivity to each point in the plane source decreases according to the inverse square law, thus leading to a constant counting rate at each point in the detector.

Equation (2.12) implies that for one collimator $R^2 P_0$ is constant. This helps to visualise the relationship between P_0 and the resolution index in Eq. (2.9) for different distances z, namely that P_0 is inversely proportional to R^2. Also from Eq. (2.11) the peak values of the line spread functions will be proportional to P_0/a and hence inversely proportional to R. Of course, once we introduce an attenuating medium, there will be an additional $\exp(-\mu z)$ factor where μ is the effective attenuation coefficient of the gamma rays in the medium, usually taken as unit density material to simulate human muscle tissue. Hence, a knowledge of the point spread function in absolute terms should specify completely the resolution and sensitivity of the system. In practice the line spread function tends to be measured experimentally for a series of values of z or depths in a tissue equivalent medium. Point, line and plane sensitivity measurements are all influenced by the choice of energy window which needs careful calibration.

The point spread function represents the variation in sensitivity from point to point and may be used to refine further the mathematical model of the imaging process. In our initial assumptions leading to Eq. (2.1), the gamma ray flux was obtained from straight line integrals. The sensitivity factor k converted the gamma ray flux to count rate per unit area of detector. If we represent the distributions of activity in the patient by the function $g(x, y, z)$, with units of activity per unit volume, then the count rate per unit area over the detector surface $D(x, y)$ is given by a convolution of the point spread function with the distribution $g(x, y, z)$, i.e., we have finally

$$D(x,y) = \int \int \int PSF(x - x', y - y', z)g(x', y', z)\, dx'\, dy' \exp(-\mu z)\, dz$$

(2.13)

In addition μ may vary with position (as in a patient with different density tissues); thus the conventional radionuclide image $D(x, y)$ is an extremely complicated function of the original distribution $g(x, y, z)$. The deduction of $g(x, y, z)$ from $D(x, y)$ is the subject of reconstruction tomography, which will be discussed in Chapter 4.

As in many other branches for physics, Fourier analysis provides a useful alternative method for representing the resolving capability of an imaging device or of separate parts of the device. Readers are already probably familiar with applications of Fourier analysis in alternating current theory where, in terms of angular frequency, the output from a network $F_0(w)$ is related to the input $F_i(w)$ by the relationship

$$F_0(w) = Z_T(w)\, F_i(w)$$

(2.14)

where $Z_T(w)$ is the transfer function of the network. For example, the transfer function of a resistor R and an inductor L in series is simply its impedance, hence

$$Z_T(w) = R + jwL$$

(2.15)

An important result is obtained when the input is a unit impulse, since the standard relationship between Fourier variables (see, e.g., Stuart, 1961)

$$F_i(w) = \int_{-\infty}^{\infty} f(t) \exp(-jwt)\, dt$$

(2.16)

now becomes

$$F_i(w) = \lim_{T \to 0} \frac{1}{2T} \int_{-T}^{T} \exp(-jwt) \, dt \qquad (2.17)$$

Hence,

$$F_i(w) = 1 \qquad (2.18)$$

Thus the input spectrum $F_i(w)$ is constant (Fig. 2.9) and the output response $F_o(w)$ is simply the transfer function of the network $Z_T(w)$.

A similar approach is useful in imaging, where the Fourier transform pair are now distance x and spatial frequency f where

$$f = w'/2\pi \qquad (2.19)$$

and w' is the spatial equivalent of w. Provided that the imaging device is a

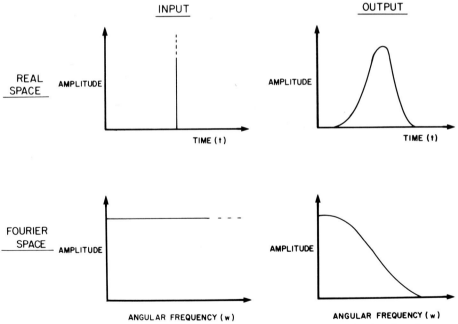

FIG. 2.9. Fourier transform of the unit impulse function. The transform is a function whose amplitude has a constant value at all angular frequencies. The shape of the output function in the Fourier domain thus gives a direct measure of how well information carried by different angular frequencies is reproduced by the network.

linear system, then by analogy, the impulse transform response is

$$G_0(f_x) = \int_{-\infty}^{\infty} \text{LSF}(x) \exp(-2\pi j f_x) \, dx \qquad (2.20)$$

This is usually an even function, so the cosine transform will suffice. After normalisation, it is termed the modulation transfer function (MTF) where

$$\text{MTF}(f_x) = \int_0^{\infty} \text{LSF}(x) \cos(2\pi f_x) \, dx \bigg/ \int_0^{\infty} \text{LSF}(x) \, dx \qquad (2.21)$$

It follows from the preceding that examination of the spatial frequencies present in the Fourier transform of the image of an impulse response gives a direct measure of how well each spatial frequency has been transmitted by a particular component of the imaging device. Since high spatial frequencies are associated with fine spatial detail, the MTF gives a direct measure of imaging performance. This approach is discussed more fully in Section 5.3.

It is important to realise that there is no more information in the MTF than in the original LSF from which it has been calculated. The benefit is simply in helping to visualise the relative effect on different spatial frequencies. If the overall imaging system can be considered as a series of individual components, each with a separate impulse response, then the overall impulse response is given by a convolution of the individual impulse responses. The overall MTF is obtained more easily, simply by multiplying the component MTFs together.

2.2 The radiopharmaceutical aspect

Radiopharmaceuticals are drugs and as such they are subject to stringent quality control both in their manufacture and use. For radionuclide imaging purposes the radiopharmaceutical will consist of an appropriate compound, which will be metabolised by or incorporated into the human tissue to be studied. In order to image its *in vivo* distribution, the compound will be labelled with a suitable radionuclide. The patient will suffer least if the radiopharmaceutical can be administered orally or intravenously, avoiding the trauma of more invasive procedures such as intra-arterial or intra-thecal injection. The choice of radionuclide will be made on the basis of suitable emission and half-life, while the compound will be chosen for appropriate biochemical, physiological or pharmacological properties. The practicalities of cost and convenience must also be

considered, and a compromise may be essential. If the biological properties of a particular compound are good and result in high selective
uptake in the target tissue, this may outweigh poor physical qualities of the
radionuclide required to label the compound.

2.2.1 Type of emission and half-life

Radiation dose to the patient must be kept to a minimum, so radionuclides
which deposit the least amount of energy in the patient for a given photon
yield should be preferred. Decay by isomeric transition or electron capture
can ideally fulfill this requirement. However, some radionuclides which
undergo beta decay accompanied by a high photon yield have proved
useful, and positron emitting radionuclides offer the unique annihilation
photons for coincidence counting methods.

The effect of photon energy on detectability was illustrated in Fig. 2.2.
For practical reasons the useful energy range can be considered as
50–511 keV. At the lower-energy end of this range the gamma rays are
excessively attenuated within the patient, while at the higher end collimator penetration becomes excessive.

The half-life of the radionuclide is also fundamental in determining
radiation dose to the patient. Unless the compound is excreted, exhaled or
otherwise removed rapidly from the body, very small quantities of
long-lived radionuclides can give a significant radiation dose to individual
organs and to the whole body. In general, therefore, the shortest half-life
possible is required, consistent with any necessary time delay to allow
localisation of the compound in the tissues of interest and the time required
to perform the imaging measurements. A half-life of 0.693 times the time
required to complete the study has been suggested as optimum in order to
maximise information with minimum radiation exposure to the patient.
Actual times required to complete the study may range from under one
minute to several days. Half-lives of under 12 h imply costly on-site
production or daily delivery to maintain a ready supply. Fortunately
several useful, relatively short-lived radionuclides are available as daughter
products of a longer-lived parent, the "radionuclide generator".

2.2.2 Radionuclides

There are three sources of radionuclides used for the preparation of
radiopharmaceuticals: the nuclear reactor, the cyclotron and the radionuclide generator.

2.2.2.1 The nuclear reactor

Nuclear reactors can produce radionuclides through neutron capture and fission reactions. Specific target elements can be subjected to (n, γ), (n, p) or (n, α) reactions. The targets either may be fixed in special irradiation positions or be brought into the reactor as mobile targets in a pneumatic system. The neutron activation process does not convert all the atoms of the target material into the desired radionuclide, and it will not be possible to separate chemically unreacted target from the radioactive product as the nuclides are of the same element. This unchanged target material is called "carrier".

Fission is the process of splitting a heavy nuclide into two fragments of approximately similar mass. If a target of a heavy element $(Z > 92)$ is inserted into the reactor core, fission will occur when the target absorbs thermal neutrons. Most fission products have atomic numbers in the range 42–56. As they are isotopes of different elements, they can be separated by appropriate chemical methods. The radionuclides produced by fission are generally carrier-free and are available at high specific activities. The most common nucleus for fission processes is 235-uranium (235-U), which is used for the production of 131-iodine (131-I), 133-xenon (133-Xe) and 99-molybdenum (99-Mo).

2.2.2.2 The cyclotron

Another way to make radioactive nuclei is to bombard stable nuclei with energetic charged particles such as protons, deuterons and alpha particles from the cyclotron. Such radionuclides are usually "proton rich" and decay by positron emission or electron capture (e.g., 123-I, 201-Tl and 18-F). The chemical properties of the target and the product will not be the same since they are different elements. The radionuclide will, therefore, be carrier-free, but side reactions may give rise to radionuclide impurities. With the development of compact medical cyclotrons and good positron imaging devices, more use is being made of the ultrashort-lived radioisotopes of the biologically important elements carbon, nitrogen and oxygen. These radionuclides can be readily incorporated into pharmaceuticals by direct substitution for their non-radioactive counterparts.

2.2.2.3 The radionuclide generator

A convenient source of short-lived radionuclides is provided by several natural decay chains in which a parent radionuclide with relatively long half-life decays to a short-lived daughter. The parent–daughter mixture, adsorbed on a suitable material, forms the basis of the generator system.

With appropriate differences in chemical behaviour between parent and daughter elements, the latter can be separated by a simple elution procedure and the daughter radionuclide then builds up again until transient equilibrium is reestablished. At this equilibrium the daughter radionuclide appears to decay with the same half-life as the parent. A further elution yields a fresh supply of the pure daughter radionuclide when required.

The 99-molybdenum (99-Mo)–99m-technetium (99m-Tc) system overshadows all others in importance for routine nuclear medicine to date.

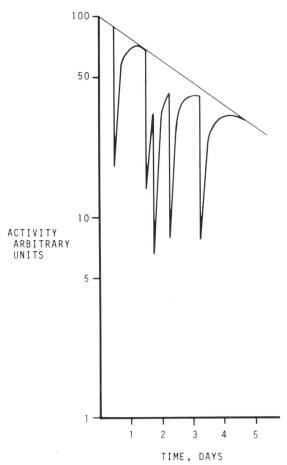

FIG. 2.10. Thin line showing the amount of 99m-Tc activity available from a 99-Mo generator. The available activity decays with a half-life identical to that of 99-Mo. The thick line shows the growth of 99m-Tc after elutions.

99-Molybdenum has a half-life of 2.8 days. It decays to 99-Tc either directly (in 13% of disintegrations) or indirectly through the metastable radionuclide 99m-Tc (87% of disintegrations). 99m-Technetium is an extremely useful radionuclide, particularly for gamma camera imaging. The isomeric transition to the ground state 99-Tc results in a high yield of virtually monoenergetic 140-keV photons, and the half-life of 6 h is almost ideal for the majority of static routine imaging investigations although a shorter half-life would be desirable for some dynamic studies. A wide range of pharmaceuticals that can be easily labelled with technetium has been developed.

In the generator, 99-Mo is adsorbed to the upper part of a small chromatographic column filled with high grade alumina (Al_2O_3). As the parent 99-Mo decays, the activity of the daughter 99m-Tc on the column will grow until a maximum is reached after approximately four 99m-Tc half-lives (24 h). At this point equilibrium is reached, the decay of 99m-Tc matching its generation from 99-Mo. The result is a supply of 99m-Tc decaying at the same rate as the 99-Mo. The 99m-Tc does not bind to the column material and can be separated by passing 0.9% saline solution through the column, the 99-Mo remaining fixed to the alumina. When sterile solutions and aseptic techniques are used, the eluate will be ready for use immediately as sodium pertechnetate. After elution, the 99m-Tc activity will start to grow again. Elution may be carried out if needed before equilibrium is again reached; the amount of 99m-Tc then available will depend on the time elapsed since the last elution (Fig. 2.10).

2.2.3 Labelling

A radionuclide which is ideal for imaging is of little value if it cannot be incorporated into a suitable compound or chemical carrier with the desired biological behaviour. To avoid any adverse reaction in the patient, the final material must be sterile (radiopharmaceuticals are not self-sterilising), pyrogen-free and at a suitable pH, with no toxic or other side effects. Particularly with the short-lived radionuclides, the chemical labelling methods should be simple and quick. The final product must be stable and have high chemical purity.

Radiochemical purity is defined as the proportion of the total radioactivity present in the desired chemical form in the radiopharmaceutical. A number of analytical methods are used to determine the radiochemical impurities, e.g., chromatography. Radionuclide purity is the proportion of radioactivity due to the desired radionuclide in the total radioactivity measured. It must be sufficiently high to avoid any excessive radiation dose to the patient from long-lived contaminants. The radionuclide purity can be assessed using gamma spectroscopy. The specific activity is the ratio of the particular radionuclide to the total mass of the element present. It should be known in order to evaluate possible effects on the incorporation of the element into the radiopharmaceutical, or its biological uptake or clearance in the patient.

In isotopic labelling, the radionuclide replaces an atom of the same element in the compound, forming an isomer. In a nonisotopic labelled compound an atom has been replaced by a radionuclide of a different element. These compounds are not isomers and it should not be taken for granted that their biological and chemical characteristics will be identical to the original.

The uptake of the radiopharmaceutical into the target tissue depends on a number of mechanisms, such as simple diffusion, adsorption, phagocytosis, active cellular transport and ion exchange. The following section gives examples of the many different compounds and methods of studying tissues through radionuclide imaging.

2.2.4   Practical compounds and applications

A wide variety of compounds has evolved, and the manufacture and supply of radiopharmaceuticals is now a major industry. The examples below are not intended to be exhaustive but simply illustrate the many different uptake mechanisms that have been utilised in order to visualise internal organs of the body.

2.2.4.1   The blood pool

The passage of a bolus of intravenously injected radiopharmaceutical, such as 99m-Tc pertechnetate, through the chambers of the heart can be recorded as a dynamic study using the gamma camera and computer. A rapid sequence of images is required for the "first-pass study", and the bolus injection requires a high radioactive concentration so that as small a volume of liquid as possible is injected. The study is completed within 30 sec or so; intra-cardiac shunts can be detected and quantified, and left or right ventricular function can be measured (Berger *et al*, 1980). Ultrashort half-life radionuclides are ideal for these investigations because of the rapid physical decay of activity. The generator-produced 195m-gold, with a half-life of 30.5 sec, is currently likely to replace 99m-Tc in the specialised cardiac centres—the study can be repeated within a few minutes on a virtually zero background, e.g., to obtain views from a different angle, or with the patient exercising.

Longer-term studies on the blood pool are performed using 99m-Tc labelled red blood cells. The patient's own red cells can be tagged *in vivo* by injecting 99m-Tc pertechnetate solution approximately 30 minutes after an intravenous injection of stannous pyrophosphate ($10-20$ μg stannous ion/kg body weight). Again the aim of the study is usually to investigate cardiac ventricular function and wall motion. By using the patient's electro-cardiogram to time the acquisition of photons, images can be built up over several minutes, each image representing a discrete fraction of the cardiac cycle (multiple-gated acquisition). The sequence of images, stored by computer, can then be analysed to assess regional wall movement, ventricular volumes and ejection rates (Berger *et al.*, 1980).

Labelled red cells may also be used to detect and localise sites of intra-abdominal bleeding or arterio-venous malformations (Miskowiak *et al.*, 1981).

2.2.4.2 *Suspensions of radioactive labelled particles*

These have proved useful for studying the lungs, the reticuloendothelial system (liver, spleen and bone marrow) and the lymphatic system. The compounds can be subdivided into four groups:

- (i)   macroaggregated particles,
- (ii) microspheres,
- (iii) microaggregated particles and
- (iv) millimicrospheres.

The difference between the first two products and the last two is, as the names indicate, in particle size. This differentiates the diagnostic uses of the products. There is no exact division but, as a guideline, macroaggregates and microspheres have a mean particle diameter greater than 1 μm. Aggregates are normally produced by denaturing a solution of human serum albumin. The mean particle size depends on the conditions of the denaturing process, such as temperature and pH. Today the pharmaceutical is supplied as a "freeze-dried preparation kit" containing prefabricated albumin particles, a dry powder in a sterile vial. The particles also contain a reducing agent which will take part in the formation of the complex of albumin particles and 99m-Tc when the eluate from a 99m-Tc generator is added to the vial.

Microspheres are small spherical particles also produced by denaturing albumin. They are more robust and can be sorted according to particle size by "sieving" after production. They are also supplied as a freeze-dried preparation kit.

Macroaggregated albumin and microspheres are used for lung perfusion studies. The particle size should be between 10 and 100 μm, ideally with a mean diameter of approximately 30–40 μm. After intravenous injection the particles are transported with the blood to the lungs and are distributed in proportion to the pulmonary blood flow, being trapped by the smallest capillaries in the vascular network of the lungs. The number of particles injected is such that only a minor fraction of the smallest blood vessels will be closed and the study will not be dangerous to the patient. The particles are biodegradable, being metabolised by the body, and after a few hours normal blood flow is restored to the lung tissue. The technique is used mainly for the detection of pulmonary embolism, which shows up as a "cold spot" on the lung images, (Fig. 2.11) (Moser *et al.*, 1971).

When injected intravenously the microaggregated albumin and milli-microspheres can be used to study the reticuloendothelial system (RES). If

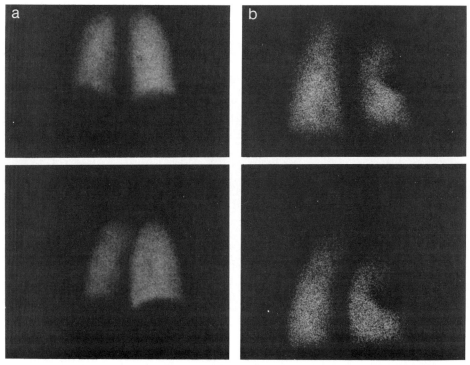

FIG. 2.11. Lung images produced with 99m-Tc macroaggregated human serum albumin. The upper pair of images is a posterior view and the lower pair a posterior oblique view. Normal images (a) show a uniform distribution of the radiopharmaceutical while the pulmonary emboli produce areas having little or no uptake (b). (Courtesy of Dr. F. W. Smith, Aberdeen Royal Infirmary.)

the particles are less than 1 μm they will pass through the pulmonary circulation and will be mainly taken up by the phagocytic cells in the RES; 90% of these cells are located in the liver and the remainder in the spleen and bone marrow. Images can thus yield significant clinical information about the structure and function of these tissues—metastatic disease or other pathology can be detected as cold spots due to the replacement of the normal cells by disease processes, (Fig. 2.12) (Braunstein and Song, 1975).

When injected into the patient via a lymph duct, the microaggregates or millimicrospheres will diffuse and enable visualisation of the patency of the lymphatic system, (Dworkin, 1982).

The disadvantage with the aggregated particles is that their shape and size are not well defined. Microspheres, as their name implies, can be made with a very narrow particle size distribution. However, at present, aggregates have a faster rate of biodegradation and are considerably less expensive than microspheres.

2.2.4.3 Ion exchange

The absence of a suitable radioisotope of calcium led to the development of phosphate complexes, such as methylene diphosphonate, for bone imaging. The first step in the localisation of these bone imaging agents is diffusion from blood into the extracellular fluid. The porous mineralised surface of the bones is surrounded by this fluid, and the phosphate complexes fix rapidly to the solid phase of the bone by ion exchange and inclusion into the hydroxyapatite lattice. The complexes are usually labelled with 99m-Tc, again in a one-step procedure, the pharmaceutical being supplied as a freeze-dried powder in a sterile vial. The concentration of radioactivity in bone will be highest where there is increased bone activity and blood flow, for instance in areas of healing bone or areas with primary or metastatic tumours (Fig. 2.13) (Pabst and Langhammer, 1977).

201-Thallium as thallous chloride is concentrated in the myocardium actively by the so-called sodium/potassium pump. Even though the thallium ion is not a true potassium analogue, its biological distribution is very similar to potassium (for which there is no suitable radioisotope). By using this radiopharmaceutical it is possible to distinguish between infarcted myocardium, ischaemic myocardium and myocardium with normal blood flow (Ashburn and Tubau, 1980).

2.2.4.4 Active transport

Iodide administered orally or intravenously will be taken up actively in the thyroid gland and used to produce thyroid hormones. Sodium iodide

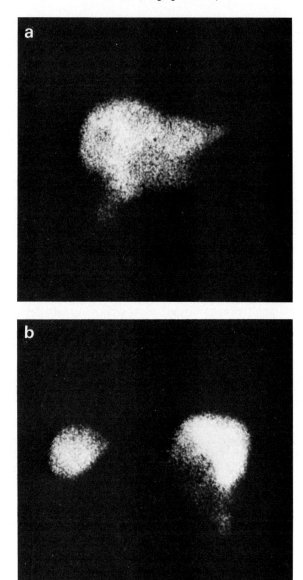

FIG. 2.12. Abnormalities in this liver study show as areas of reduced or absent uptake of the radiopharmaceutical: (a) anterior view and (b) posterior view. In (b) the area of uptake on the left is the spleen. (Courtesy of Dr. F. W. Smith, Aberdeen Royal Infirmary.)

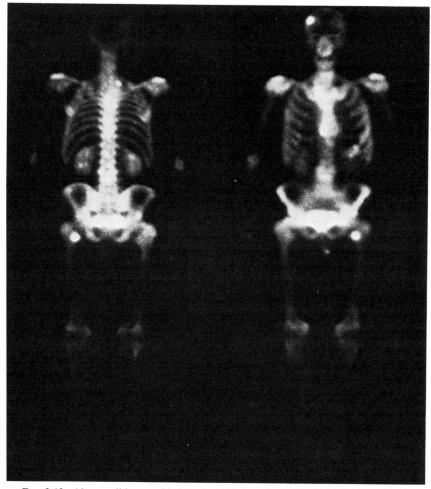

FIG. 2.13. Abnormalities on this bone scan appear as well defined areas of increased uptake. There are such areas in the skull, throughout the spine and pelvis and in the left femoral head. (Courtesy of Dr. F. W. Smith, Aberdeen Royal Infirmary.)

solution labelled with 131-I, or more recently with 123-I, can be used to study the process of thyroid hormone formation, storage and metabolism. Primary and metastatic malignant tumours and other lesions of the gland can be detected by their differential concentration of the radioactive tracer (Fig. 2.14).

99m-Technetium-iminodiacetic acid (IDA) derivatives use the principle of active transport to study the function of the liver/gall bladder system.

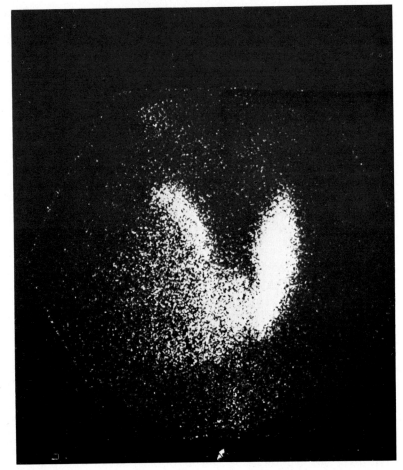

FIG. 2.14. Lobe on the left of the thyroid gland shows a large, diffuse area of reduced uptake. (Courtesy of Dr. F. W. Smith, Aberdeen Royal Infirmary.)

These compounds are actively taken up by the polygonal cells in the liver and secreted as bile through the gall bladder system into the gut (Fig. 2.15) (Nicholson *et al.*, 1980). The pharmaceutical can again be supplied as a freeze-dried powder in a sterile vial.

Iodohippuric acid (Hippuran) is actively secreted by the renal tubules and partially reabsorbed by the blood. Hippuran labelled with radioiodine (preferably 123-I) is thus used to study kidney function, (Fig. 2.16) (O'Reilly *et al.*, 1979).

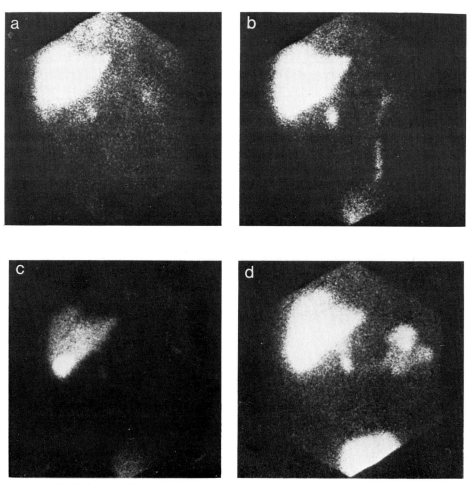

FIG. 2.15. Study of the hepato-biliary system. (a) and (b) In the first 15 min of the study, material is mainly concentrated in the liver with a little being cleared by the kidneys. (c) By 20 min, activity has passed into the gall bladder. (d) Later on, material has also gone into the duodenum and intestines. (Courtesy of Dr. F. W. Smith, Aberdeen Royal Infirmary.)

2.2.4.5 Radioactive gases for inhalation or injection

The noble gases xenon and krypton have radioisotopes suitable for lung ventilation studies. 133-Xenon and 127-xenon are commercially available as precalibrated doses and are diluted with air in a ventilation circuit. The patient breathes from the circuit and an image is taken once the gas has been inhaled for long enough to fill the ventilating volume of the lung. The

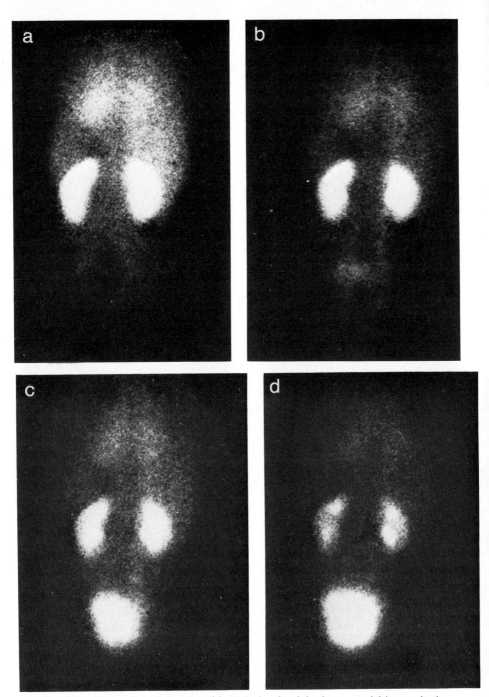

Fig. 2.16. Study of renal function. (a) At 1 min after injection, material is seen in the kidneys and a little in the heart and background tissue. (b) By 4 min, material has moved into the renal pelvis and a little has drained into the bladder. In this normal study, continuing drainage from the kidneys and bladder filling can be seen in the images taken at 12 min (c) and 20 min (d). (Courtesy of Dr. F. W. Smith, Aberdeen Royal Infirmary.)

circuit is then adjusted so that the xenon is exhaled and only air inhaled. A series of images taken during this time shows the washout of gas from the lungs. Areas of lung showing poor ventilation or slow gas clearance can be identified (Moser *et al.*, 1971).

81m-Krypton is an ultrashort-lived gas (half-life = 13 sec) and is available from an 81-Rb generator by eluting with air which is then piped directly to the patient. The resulting image shows regional ventilatory rate (Goris and Daspit, 1978).

Xenon dissolved in sterile saline solution has been used to study both lung perfusion and blood flow. The gas is removed in its first passage through the lungs, as it is more soluble in air than in blood.

2.2.4.6 Compartmental localisation

The body has several well-separated compartments. When a radioactive tracer is introduced into a compartment, it will not leave the compartment under normal circumstances. Thus, the tracer can be used to measure parameters within the compartment such as flow dynamics or volume estimation.

In radionuclide cisternography, the radiopharmaceutical is introduced intrathecally (via lumbar puncture) into the cerebro-spinal fluid (CSF). Thus, the production, distribution and reabsorption of this fluid can be studied (Harbert, 1971). 169-Ytterbium, 99m-technetium or 111-indium labelled diethylenetriamine penta-acetic acid (DTPA) is currently used.

Brain tumours and vascular lesions of the brain are examples of conditions which lead to a change or breakdown of the normal blood–brain barrier. Many of the radiopharmaceuticals used in blood-pool studies will be able to cross the barrier at these damaged sites and, thus, permit visualisation of these areas (Fig. 2.17) (Front, 1978).

2.2.4.7 Tumour-specific compounds

No pharmaceutical presently in use is totally tumour-specific, i.e., incorporated into tumour tissue only. Such products would be very helpful in the search for early stages of primary and metastatic tumours and for therapy purposes. 67-Gallium citrate and 111-indium bleomycin complexes have been shown to localise in some tumour sites, but imaging is confounded by considerable uptake in other tissues of the body. A wide range of anti-tumour agents is available for labelling and methods have been developed for antibodies, hormones and other substances that specifically attach to malignant cells. The introduction of cloning technology makes it possible to produce, *in vitro*, large amounts of pure antibodies from one single cell. Such monoclonal antibodies labelled with radionuclides may prove to be useful tumour markers (Sfakianakis and DeLand, 1982).

a   b

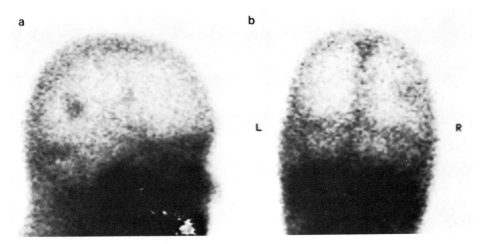

Fig. 2.17. Brain scan showing an area of increased uptake positioned posteriorly in the right lateral view (a) and superficially in the posterior view (b). There is a second, smaller lesion situated slightly anteriorly to the first. These appearances suggest metastases.

2.2.5 Rate of uptake and clearance

For many radiopharmaceuticals localisation in the target tissues is related to the rate of plasma clearance after administration. Variations in distribution and clearance occur according to particle size, permeabilities, excretion rates, etc. For static imaging the optimum time to image the target tissue is a compromise between target to non-target concentration ratio and physical decay of the radionuclide. An appropriate signal to noise ratio will thus be seen to increase as the radionuclide is concentrated in the target and cleared from the background. However, since this clearance is never complete, a maximum will be reached, after which the SNR will be diminished by radioactive decay. The optimum time will correspond to the maximum.

The disappearance of a radiopharmaceutical from a biological system will depend both on the decay of the radionuclide, characterised by the physical half-life t_p, and the biological half-life t_b. The biological half-life is the time required to eliminate half of the pharmaceutical by the regular elimination processes of the body. If the biological disappearance follows an exponential law, as it will do if behaviour approximates a one-compartment model, then the effective half-life of the radiopharmaceutical (which includes loss of activity due to both physical decay and biological elimination is represented by t_e, where

$$1/t_e = (1/t_p) + (1/t_b) \qquad (2.22)$$

Radiopharmaceuticals should have a short effective half-life, ideally not much longer than the time needed to complete the study, as was stated earlier for the physical half-life. However, a radiopharmaceutical incorporating a radionuclide of very long physical half-life could still be a good agent if the biological half-life was short.

Other drugs may be administered to the patient as well as the radiopharmaceutical, either to enhance uptake in the target tissue or to reduce uptake in the non-target tissue, or to accelerate elimination from the body. This may help to maximise information with minimum radiation exposure to the patient.

References

Ashburn, W. L. and Tubau, J. (1980). Myocardial perfusion imaging in ischaemic heart diseases. *Radio. Clin. N. Am.* **18,** 467–486.

Berger, H.J., Gottschalk, A. and Zabet, B. L. (1980). Radionuclide assessment of left and right ventricular function. *Radiol. Clin. N. Am.* **18,** 441–445.

Braunstein, P. and Song, C. S. (1975). The uses and limitations of radioisotopes in the investigation of gastrointestinal diseases. *Am. J. Dig. Dis.* **20,** 53–89.

Dworkin, H. J. (1982). Potential for lymphoscintigraphy *J Nucl. Med.* **23,** 936–938.

Front, D. (1978). Scintigraphic assessment of vascularity and brain-tissue barrier of human brain tumour. *J. Neurol., Neurosurg. Psychiatry* **41,** 18–23.

Goris, M. and Daspit, S. (1978). Krypton-81m. *Prog. Nucl. Med.* **5,** 69–92.

Harbert, J. C. (1971). Radionuclide cisternography. *Semin. Nucl. Med.* **1,** 90–106.

Miskowiak, J., Nielson, S. L. and Munch, O. (1981). Scintigraphic diagnosis of gastrointestinal bleeding with 99m-Tc labelled bloodpool agents. *Radiology* **141,** 499–504.

Moser, K. M., Guisan, M., Cuomo, A. and Ashburn, W. L. (1971). Differentiation of pulmonary vascular from parenchymal diseases by ventilation/perfusion scintigraphy. *Ann. Intern. Med.* **75,** 597–605.

Nicholson, R. W., Hastings, D. L., Testa, H. J. and Torrance, B. (1980). HIDA scanning in gall-bladder disease. *Br. J. Radiol.* **53,** 878–882.

O'Reilly, P. H., Shields, R. A. and Testa, H. J. (1979). "Nuclear Medicine in Urology and Nephrology". Butterworth, London.

Pabst, H. W. and Langhammer, H. (1977). Detection and differential diagnosis of bone lesions by scintigraphy. *Eur. J. Nucl. Med.* **2,** 261–268.

Sfakianakis, G. N. and DeLand, F. H. (1982). Radioimmunodiagnosis and radioimmunotherapy. *J. Nucl. Med.* **23,** 840–850.

Stuart, R. D. (1961). "An Introduction to Fourier Analysis". Methuen, London.

Tsui, B. M. W., Metz, C. E. and Beck, R. N. (1983). Optimum detector resolution for discriminating between tumour uptake distributions in scintigraphy. *Phys. Med. Biol.* **28,** 775–778.

Chapter 3

Physical Principles of
in vivo Imaging Systems

3.1 Introduction

The first attempt to image the *in vivo* distribution of a radiopharmaceutical was based on point-by-point measurements made with a Geiger–Müller counter positioned by hand over a grid placed against the thyroid. Such a method was obviously time-consuming and, while feasible for a small organ like the thyroid gland, offered little potential for larger organs.

The rectilinear scanner developed as an automated version of this technique, but the sequential nature of image formation proved to be a severe drawback particularly when short exposure times were needed, as in dynamic studies. This problem was overcome by the gamma camera which has now superseded the rectilinear scanner, where supporting facilities are adequate, for all but a few specialised applications.

The camera itself suffers from several limitations, and proposals for alternative devices will be considered in Chapter 7. Unfortunately, few of these devices have shown any commercial potential and the camera remains the main imaging instrument.

In addition to scanners and cameras, the whole-body counter also plays an important role in nuclear medicine. Although it has very limited imaging capability, it can provide some information on the distribution of low levels of radioactive material, particularly over long periods of time.

3.2 The rectilinear scanner

The rectilinear scanner was the first instrument to image effectively a distribution of gamma-emitting radionuclide within the body (Cassen *et al.*, 1951; Mayneord *et al.*, 1951). It is simply a scintillation counter, collimated so as to record the count rate from a well-defined volume beneath it, the image being built up by moving the detector in a raster pattern over the patient. The image thus consists of intensity signals derived from the detector and spatial co-ordinates representing the position of the gantry carrying the detector. A dual-headed scanner is shown in Fig. 3.1, together with a schematic diagram of the instrument.

3.2.1 Detector and collimator

Typically, the detector is a NaI(Tl) crystal 8–13 cm in diameter and 5 cm thick fitted with a lead shield and collimator to form an efficient detector for gamma rays of energy up to 500 keV. While scanners could be designed to image gamma rays of even higher energies, difficulties arise in mechanically moving the very heavy collimators which would be needed.

As positional information is derived from the location of the detector, spatial resolution and sensitivity are predominantly determined by the design of the collimator and the dimensions of the scintillation crystal. The purpose of the collimator is to restrict the field of view of the detector to the small volume of material immediately beneath it. This is achieved by using an array of tapered holes focussed on a point several centimetres in front of the collimator face, thus allowing a high proportion of those gamma rays emitted from the region around the focus to be detected (Fig. 3.2).

For gamma rays of energy less than 150 keV, penetration of the lead septa between the holes can be ignored and performance of the focussed collimator may be predicted solely from geometry. Both resolution and sensitivity can be measured from the impulse response, i.e., the image produced when a point or line source of radioactivity is scanned (Chapter 2). For practical reasons (Tyson and Amtey, 1978) resolution is usually measured from the LSF.

Using the notation of Fig. 3.2, the radius of the field of view R_F in the focal plane of a focussed collimator is

$$R_F = 2rf/t \qquad (3.1)$$

The FWHM of the PSF is approximately equal to 0.8 R_F.

The sensitivity of a collimator can be expressed by its geometric efficiency, the proportion of gamma rays emitted from a source which,

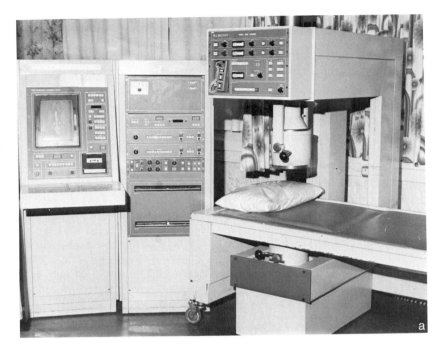

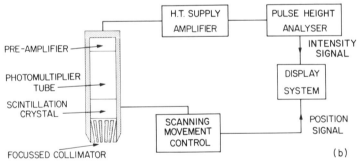

FIG. 3.1. (a) Dual-headed rectilinear scanner and (b) schematic diagram of the scanner.

according to the geometry of the collimator's construction, will reach the detector. No account is taken of scatter, detector efficiency and pulse height analysis, so it will differ numerically from experimentally determined sensitivity. Sensitivity is discussed in detail in Chapter 5.

Efficiency has been defined for cases when the source is either a uniform plane of activity covering the collimator's field of view or a point. In the former case, as all the collimator holes will be flooded with gamma rays,

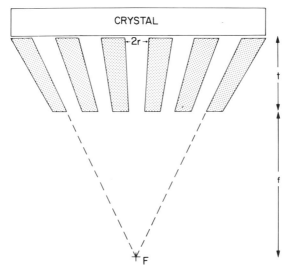

Fig. 3.2. Cross-section through a focussed collimator. The collimator is of length t and has holes of radius r focussed to a point F a distance f from the front face of the collimator.

changes in the distance of the source from the face of the collimator will not alter the number of gamma rays reaching the detector. The value for efficiency will, however, change if the field of view, and hence the total activity seen by the collimator, varies. One alternative definition for efficiency uses the ratio of detected count rate to activity per unit area in the plane, which makes geometric efficiency independent of source–collimator separation. Such a measure of efficiency has units of area. To avoid confusion this definition of efficiency will not be used.

Plane sources give the average efficiency of the collimator. For certain collimators, efficiency varies across the field of view as well as with source–collimator distance. In these cases the point source is more useful as it allows efficiency to be expressed as a function of spatial position. For this reason both the plane and point source efficiency will be used in this book, the former being defined as

$$E = \frac{\text{photon flux reaching detector}}{\substack{\text{activity per unit area in the plane source} \\ \times \text{ field of view of collimator}}} \tag{3.2}$$

and for the point source

$$E^{\mathrm{P}} = \frac{\text{photon flux reaching detector}}{\text{activity in the point source}} \tag{3.3}$$

For the focussed collimator, its geometric efficiency as measured with a plane source is given by (Beck, 1964)

$$E_F = Nr^2/16(f+t)^2 \tag{3.4}$$

where the collimator has N circular holes.

A comparison of Eqs. (3.1) and (3.4) shows the conflicting requirements for good spatial resolution and high efficiency. For a fixed value of N, increasing hole radius r improves efficiency but worsens resolution.

Table 3.1 gives the performance parameters for a typical medium-sensitivity collimator designed for use at low energies. Resolution in the focal plane is 1.2 cm ($0.8R_F$) while the efficiency is 0.0055. This low value for efficiency emphasises how few of the emitted gamma rays are actually used by a collimated detector to form the image.

When imaging higher-energy radionuclides, septal penetration must be taken into account and the preceding equations modified (Beck, 1964; MacIntyre et al., 1969).

The variation of the PSF with distance from the collimator face is shown in Fig. 3.3. For a rectilinear scanner the PSF simply shows how point sensitivity (not efficiency, as these are experimental measurements) varies with lateral position. As mentioned in Chapter 2, plane sensitivity is proportional to the area under the PSF and, for the measurements made in air, is independent of source–collimator distance. When tissue equivalent material is present, attenuation results in sensitivity being highest when the source is closest to the collimator.

As expected, Fig. 3.3 shows that resolution is best in the focal plane but deteriorates for points nearer to or further from the collimator.

As organs to be imaged are frequently thick and the depth of any abnormality is not known in advance, so-called depth-independent collimators have been designed specifically to minimise the rate of loss of resolution, i.e., to increase the depth of focus (Lakshmanan et al., 1975).

Sensitivity can be increased, without affecting resolution, if the number of holes N can be increased, but this requires the area of the face of the scintillation crystal to be increased which unfortunately leads to a drop in the depth of focus. This small depth of focus is, however, an advantage when producing tomographic images (Chapter 4).

TABLE 3.1. Design parameters for a medium sensitivity, low energy, focussed collimator.

Number of holes (N)	Hole radius (r), cm	Length of hole (t), cm	Focal length (f), cm	Radius of field of view (R_F), cm	Geometric efficiency (E_F)
55	0.7	8.5	9	1.5	0.0055

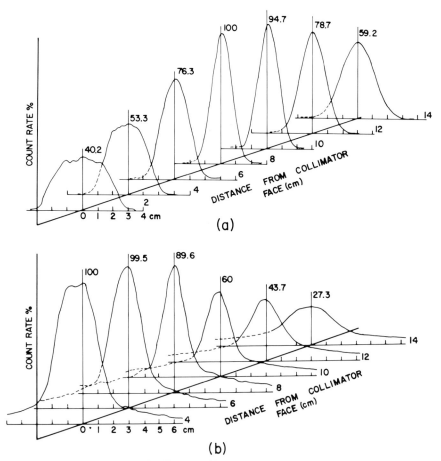

FIG. 3.3. PSF of a focussed collimator of focal length 9 cm at different distances from the collimator face. (a) Measurements made in air. (b) Measurements made in MIX D tissue equivalent wax.

3.2.2   Pulse height analyser

Signals from the detector pass through a pulse height analyser to discriminate against radiation scattered into the detector from outside the field of view, scatter which would otherwise contribute to a degrading and unwanted background signal. However, the limited energy resolution of the NaI(Tl) crystal when used as a scintillation detector, typically 10–15% at 140 keV, and the relative predominance of small angle Compton scatter lead to the presence of much scattered radiation within the photo-peak region, typically about 30% of the photons being scattered. The choice of an optimum window setting is a compromise between good sensitivity, which requires a wide window, and good spatial resolution, for which a narrow window is best. Although attempts have been made to define the best window (Atkins *et al.*, 1976), much work still remains to be done. For 99m-Tc it is generally accepted that an energy window of 120–160 keV leads to a good compromise between sensitivity and spatial resolution.

3.2.3 Display

The simplest intensity signal from the scanner is one taken from a count-rate meter. In one form of display this signal is used to determine the frequency with which a mechanical tapper arm hits an inked ribbon onto a sheet of paper. By moving the tapper unit over the sheet in synchrony with the detector, an image is produced in which density is proportional to count rate. A similar principle is employed in the photo-scan display (Kuhl *et al.*, 1962) but here the count rate modulates the brightness of a light spot moved over a sheet of X-ray film. A third variant uses the rate meter signal to position a multicolour inking ribbon in an electromechanical colour printer to produce an instant colour-coded image (Mallard and Peachey, 1959).

In a modern display, the number of gamma rays detected in scanning a predetermined distance is stored in a digital memory and displayed on a TV monitor as a pixel (picture element), coded either as grey shades or colour. While not giving an immediate hard copy image, it does allow simple image manipulations to be performed.

3.3 The gamma camera

In contrast to the sequential imaging process used in rectilinear scanning, the gamma camera, first described by Anger (1958), employs parallel sampling of the data, gamma rays from all parts of the patient within the field of view being acquired for the whole of the exposure time. The function of the collimator is thus to form the image in the scintillation crystal, with the crystal size determining the camera's overall field of view. This design has the advantage over the scanner that, no matter how short an exposure time is used, an image from the whole of the field of view will be produced, a feature which makes the camera ideal for dynamic studies.

The camera consists of two units (Fig. 3.4a), the collimated detector mounted on a stand to allow it to be manoeuvred around the patient and the console containing pulse processing electronics and displays. A simple block diagram is given in Fig. 3.4b.

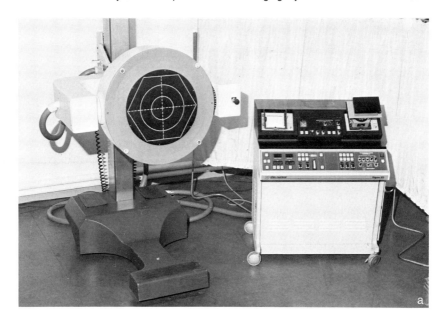

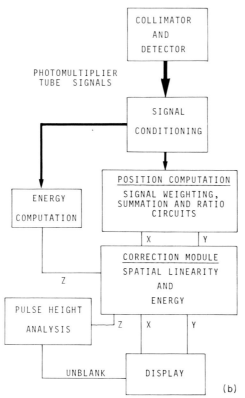

PHOTOMULTIPLIER
TUBE SIGNALS

COLLIMATOR
AND
DETECTOR

SIGNAL
CONDITIONING

POSITION COMPUTATION
SIGNAL WEIGHTING,
SUMMATION AND RATIO
CIRCUITS

ENERGY
COMPUTATION

X   Y

CORRECTION MODULE
SPATIAL LINEARITY
AND
ENERGY

Z

PULSE HEIGHT
ANALYSIS

Z   X   Y

UNBLANK   DISPLAY

(b)

FIG. 3.4. (a) Gamma camera and (b) schematic diagram of the camera.

3.3.1   The collimator

Since gamma rays are emitted isotropically, there is no inherent relationship between the position at which a gamma ray interacts with the
scintillation crystal and its point of emission in the patient. To produce an
image in the crystal, it is first necessary to use a collimator to limit the
photons detected to those travelling in an appropriate direction. A
parallel-hole collimator is used for the majority of studies, although other
types may be employed for specialised tasks.

3.3.1.1   Parallel-hole collimator

In the parallel-hole collimator the holes are perpendicular to the crystal
face (Fig. 3.5), so only gamma rays travelling in this direction will be
detected, obliquely incident gamma rays being absorbed by the lead septa
between the holes.

The spatial resolution of the collimator will depend upon the geometric
acceptance of the collimator hole with a correction applied for the small
degree of penetration of the septa by gamma rays. If resolution R_p of the
image of a point source at P (Fig. 3.5) is measured by its FWHM, then
(Anger, 1964)

$$R_p = 2r(t_e + d + c)/t_e \qquad (3.5)$$

where r is the hole radius and t_e the effective thickness of the collimator
after penetration has been taken into account (Mather, 1957)

$$t_e = t - (2/\mu) \qquad (3.6)$$

where μ is the linear attenuation coefficient for gamma rays in the
collimator material.

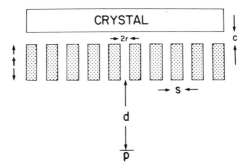

FIG. 3.5. Parallel-hole collimator.

For imaging low-energy gamma rays (about 140 keV), a minimal septa thickness of about 0.2 mm is desirable and corrugated lead foil has been used in preference to casting.

As for the rectilinear scanner collimator, the sensitivity of the collimator can be expressed by its geometric efficiency E^{P}. The geometric efficiency of the collimator is given by

$$E^{P} = \left[\frac{Kr^2}{t_e(2r + s)} \right]^2 \tag{3.7}$$

where K is a factor dependent on the shape of the holes and their pattern (Muehllehner *et al.*, 1976). For this collimator, the expression for the plane source and point source geometric efficiency is identical.

Equation (3.5) shows that resolution worsens with increasing distance from the collimator face. If attenuating material is present, then efficiency will also decrease with distance. For optimum results it is, therefore, necessary to get the patient as close to the collimator as is possible.

A comparison of Eqs. (3.5) and (3.7) shows that the conditions for high efficiency, namely thin collimators with large holes, are not consistent with those for fine resolution, so the appropriate collimator must be chosen for a particular study depending on whether resolution or count density must be optimised. The design parameters for a set of commercial collimators are shown in Table 3.2. In collimators designed for a particular energy, hole size is left unchanged and collimator thickness altered to produce high-resolution, medium- and high-sensitivity collimators. As would be expected, the resolution of each set of collimators for a particular energy is identical at the collimator face, but that for the high-sensitivity collimator degrades most rapidly with increasing distance from the collimator face.

Collimator resolution is not the only factor affecting spatial information; the camera's intrinsic resolution R_i must also be taken into account. This is a measure of the accuracy with which the image formed by the collimator in the crystal can be converted into electronic signals and will be discussed in Section 3.3.2. If the line spread functions for the collimator and the intrinsic component are gaussian, then system resolution R_s is given by the equation.

$$R_s = (R_p^2 + R_i^2)^{1/2} \tag{3.8}$$

No matter how small the collimator resolution, system resolution will be at least as large as the intrinsic resolution. Conversely, since the minimum value of the collimator resolution is limited by sensitivity, it is not worthwhile continually improving camera performance to reduce intrinsic resolution to a very low value.

TABLE 3.2. Typical design parameters for gamma camera collimators.

Type of collimator	Energy, keV	Resolution (FWHM), mm		Relative efficiency for a point source	Collimator thickness (t), mm	Number of holes	Hole radius (r), mm	Septal thickness (s), mm
		at collimator face	10 cm from collimator					
Parallel, high resolution	140	5.3	9.4	1	31.8	41000	0.75	0.2
Parallel, high sensitivity	140	5.5	13.8	3.3	17.3	41000	0.75	0.2
Parallel, high energy	400	7.3	14.7	1.2	63.5	3400	3.15	1.5
Converging	140	5.3	10	2.7[a] 4.6[b]	26.7	20000	1.2	0.2
Pinhole	140	—	3.9	0.4	—	1	1.5	—

[a] At collimator face.
[b] 10 cm from collimator face.

In clinical practice imaging will be carried out in the presence of scatter. Since at low energies it is impractical to discriminate against all scattered radiation on the basis of energy, spatial resolution will inevitably be worsened as scatter increases. Scatter effectively increases the angle of acceptance of gamma rays and will be dependent upon the distribution of the radioactivity, pulse height analyser settings and the depth of the scattering medium. Ehrhardt (1974) has shown that the effect of scatter is, however, constant for different types of collimators and he proposed that it should be simply denoted by a separate resolution component, R_{sc}. Equation (3.8) then becomes

$$R_s = (R_p^2 + R_i^2 + R_{sc}^2)^{1/2} \qquad (3.9)$$

3.3.1.2   *Converging collimator*

Although the large field of view of a modern camera is undoubtedly an advantage for imaging large organs such as the lung and the liver, in other cases, such as the brain, much of the detector surface is not being utilised. This can be rectified by using a converging collimator (Fig. 3.6) in which the holes converge towards the patient so that gamma rays diverging from

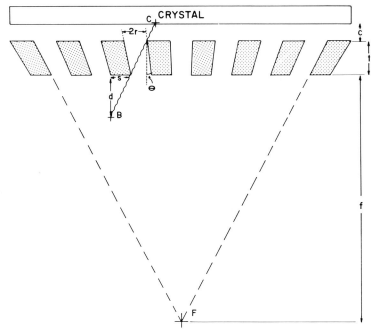

Fig. 3.6. Converging collimator with focus at *F*.

the patient are detected and an enlarged image is formed in the detector crystal. Since the intrinsic resolution relates to distances in the image plane, for a magnified image it will be reduced in inverse proportion to the magnification, e.g., a camera with intrinsic resolution of 5 mm when employed with a converging collimator producing an image twice life-size will have an effective intrinsic resolution of 2.5 mm. Converging collimators therefore provide the capability of high-resolution imaging. The resolution R_c, the FWHM measured in the object plane of a point source (B in Fig. 3.6), is given by (Moyer, 1974)

$$R_c = 2r\left(\frac{t_e + d + c}{t_e}\right)\left(\frac{1}{\cos \theta}\right)\left(1 - \frac{c + t_e/2}{f + c + t_e}\right) \tag{3.10}$$

where θ is the slant angle of that hole furthest from P through which gamma rays will just past (ray BC in Fig. 3.6). There is thus some degradation of resolution towards the edge of the field of view.

Owing to the angulation of the holes, sensitivity will also vary. For the point source at B, the geometric efficiency is

$$E_c^p = \left[\frac{Kr^2\cos \theta}{t_e(2r + s)}\right]^2 \left(\frac{f}{f - d}\right)^2 \tag{3.11}$$

Equation (3.11) is similar to that for the efficiency of a parallel hole collimator but the effective length of the angled holes is now $t_e/\cos \theta$ and the second term takes account of magnification. As θ increases towards the edge of the collimator, efficiency will decrease towards the periphery of the field of view.

The effect on efficiency of increasing source–collimator separation can be misleading. E_c^p increases as the point source is moved towards the collimator focus. Plane source efficiency, however, will decrease with increasing separation since, as mentioned earlier, the photon flux arriving at the detector remains constant while the activity seen by the collimator decreases as the field of view gets smaller.

For a source of any size, the highest photon flux will be recorded when the source just fills the collimator's field of view. In practice this increase in sensitivity with distance helps to compensate for attenuation by overlying tissue. Resolution decreases as the source moves away from the collimator, but the loss is not so severe as with the parallel-hole collimator since the intrinsic resolution of the camera is effectively decreased by the increase in image magnification.

Thus, the converging collimator offers the advantage of higher sensitivity than a parallel-hole collimator of similar resolution and less rapid degradation of resolution with depth. Its disadvantages are first, that since magnification varies with depth, it is difficult to estimate size; second, spatial distortion is produced both by the magnification effect and the variation of resolution in a plane; and finally, sensitivity varies across a plane. Brain images taken with both a parallel-hole and converging collimator are shown for comparison in Fig. 3.7. Typical performance parameters for a collimator are given in Table 3.2.

a

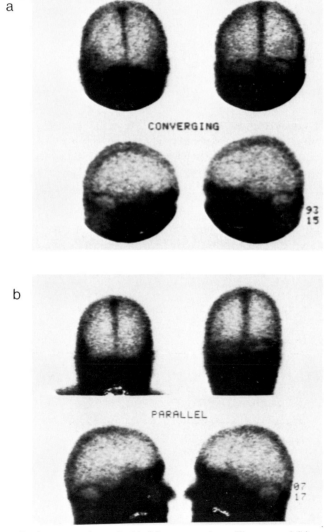

FIG. 3.7. Brain scan performed with (a) a converging collimator and (b) a parallel-hole collimator.

3.3.1.3 Diverging collimator

While converging collimators magnify the image to fill the crystal of a large field of view camera, diverging collimators (Fig. 3.8) are primarily used to minify the image of a large organ, such as the liver, so that it can be recorded in a single view on a small field of view crystal (Anger, 1958; Muehllehner, 1969).

Its resolution R_D in the object plane is given by

$$R_D = 2r\left(\frac{t_e + d + c}{t_e}\right)\left(\frac{1}{\cos\theta}\right)\left(1 + \frac{c + \frac{1}{2}t_e}{f}\right) \tag{3.12}$$

and its efficiency

$$E_D^P = \left(\frac{Kr^2\cos\theta}{t_e(2r+s)}\right)^2\left(\frac{f+t}{f+t+d}\right)^2 \tag{3.13}$$

Both efficiency and resolution deteriorate with increasing distance from the collimator face. As expected, there are similarities between the equations for R_D and R_C, and E_D^P and E_C^P, and indeed collimators have

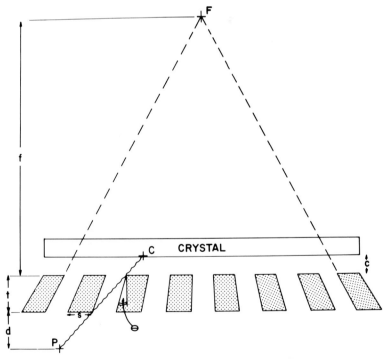

Fig. 3.8. Diverging collimator with focus at F.

been designed which when used one way round are converging and when reversed become diverging.

With large field of view cameras diverging collimators are rarely necessary, although for scanning cameras (Section 3.3.7.2) special collimators are sometimes used in which the holes diverge only in the direction transverse to the scanning motion so that the camera field of view covers the width of a patient. This is the so-called fish-tail collimator.

3.3.1.4 Pinhole collimator

In Anger's original camera the image was produced by a pinhole collimator (Fig. 3.9). This is identical to the optical pinhole except that the pinhole is made from lead and has a diameter of a few millimetres. An inverted image is formed in the crystal with a magnification t/d.

The geometric resolution R_{PH} is given by

$$R_{\text{PH}} = [(t+d)/t]2r_{\text{e}} \tag{3.14}$$

where r_{e} is the effective radius of the pinhole after allowance has been made for penetration:

$$r_{\text{e}} = r + 1/(2\mu\cot \alpha) \tag{3.15}$$

As with the converging collimator, the effective intrinsic resolution will be reduced by image magnification.

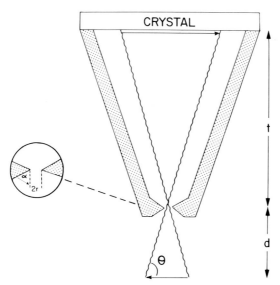

Fɪɢ. 3.9. Pinhole collimator.

So, the total resolution is given by

$$R_S = [R_{PH}^2 + (d/tR_i)^2]^{1/2} \tag{3.16}$$

The geometric efficiency E_{PH}^P is given by

$$E_{PH}^P = r^2 \sin^3 \theta / 4d^2 \tag{3.17}$$

Thus, as aperture-source distance d decreases, image size and efficiency increase and resolution improves. Increasing the pinhole size r will improve efficiency but only at the expense of resolution (Table 3.2). With increasing gamma-ray energy, penetration will increase the effective hole size and worsen resolution, but this effect can be reduced by using materials such as tungsten and platinum which have a higher μ than lead.

As magnification varies with distance, thick objects in particular will be distorted. Resolution and efficiency vary across the field of view and both comma and pincushion distortion are present. Consequently pinhole collimators are of most value for small superficial organs such as the thyroid. Figure 3.10 shows a pinhole collimator and parallel collimator view of a thyroid gland. The advantage of having a magnified image is apparent.

3.3.2   The detector

The purpose of the detector sub-system is to enable a set of electronic signals to be produced from the array of PMTs suitable for accurate computation of both the spatial location and the energy of a gamma ray interacting in the scintillation crystal. Its components are shown in Fig. 3.11.

Spatial information can be degraded in two ways. First, a series of events at the same spatial location in the crystal may produce a series of positional signals from the PMTs whose values differ from each other. Instead of a point, the image will appear as a disc. This lack of reproducibility in the computation of spatial information is known as the intrinsic resolution of the camera. Second, the computed spatial location may not represent the true position of the event, i.e., images may be spatially distorted. Such distortion is known as spatial non-linearity.

Resolution, or reproducibility, is mainly influenced by the intensity of light from the scintillation incident on the photocathodes. At low intensities the small number of photons reaching a PMT will have an intrinsic statistical variability; if N is the mean number of light photons, then the actual number received will have a standard deviation of $N^{1/2}$. For good intrinsic resolution, therefore, each PMT should receive a high light flux,

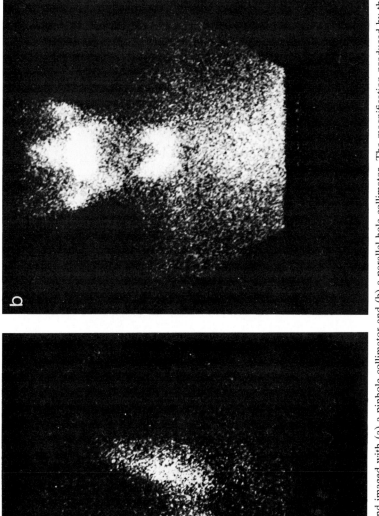

Fig. 3.10. Thyroid gland imaged with (a) a pinhole collimator and (b) a parallel-hole collimator. The magnification produced by the pinhole collimator is obvious.

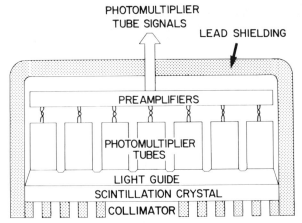

F<small>IG</small>. 3.11. Cross-section through the detector head of a gamma camera.

i.e., the solid angle subtended by the events at the photocathodes should be maximised.

Spatial linearity is optimised by sharing the light amongst many PMTs, either by increasing the distance between the PMT array and crystal or by using a large array of PMTs with small photo-cathodes. Thus, the requirement for good linearity is at variance with that for good resolution, and camera design must be aimed at producing a workable compromise.

One other factor must be taken into account, namely the sensitivity of the detector. Not only must the crystal stop most of the incident gamma rays, but to avoid loss of intrinsic resolution the photoelectric interaction must predominate. Sodium-activated cesium iodide crystals have been suggested as an alternative to NaI(Tl) since they have a higher photo-electric cross section, but as they also have a lower conversion efficiency, in practice they offer no overall advantage.

A majority of cameras use a half-inch-thick crystal which is a very efficient detector for the low-energy gamma rays of 99m-Tc, for example, but shows a rapid drop in photo-peak efficiency at higher energies (Fig. 3.12). While there is thus an apparent advantage in using a thicker crystal to improve the detection of higher-energy rays, in practice image quality will deteriorate. Primarily this is caused by differences between the distribution of light photons resulting from a gamma ray absorbed near the front surface of the scintillation crystal and that when the interaction occurs near the rear surface. The result is a degradation of linearity (Baker and Scrimger, 1967).

Second, increasing crystal thickness will increase the probability that a gamma ray will undergo multiple interactions in the crystal. A gamma ray

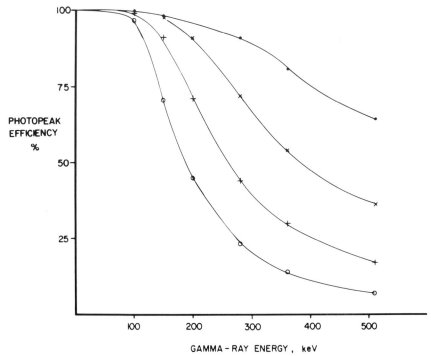

Fig. 3.12. Percentage of photo-electric interactions in an NaI(Tl) scintillation crystal. The crystal thickness is 2 in. (●), 1 in. (x), $\frac{1}{2}$ in.(+) and $\frac{1}{4}$ in. (○).

which is first Compton scattered and then absorbed by the photoelectric effect will lose the same total energy as if it had been initially absorbed. The computed position of this "scattered and absorbed" gamma ray will, however, be the centre of gravity of the series of interactions rather than the location of the first interaction and so intrinsic resolution will be degraded. In practice this effect is small and can be ignored (Anger and Davis, 1964).

With many studies now being carried out with low-energy gamma-ray emitters, there is a tendency to use crystals thinner than 13 mm ($\frac{1}{2}$ in.) to improve intrinsic resolution. For example, a 6-mm-thick crystal appears to improve intrinsic resolution by about 25% with a consequent deterioration in sensitivity of about 20% at 140 keV and a negligible loss at 80 keV (Royal *et al.*, 1979). Several cameras now use a 6-mm or 9-mm-thick crystal.

Using low-energy gamma rays will by itself degrade intrinsic resolution since such photons produce fewer light photons. Intrinsic resolution is approximately proportional to the inverse of the square root of the photon energy.

A light guide may be used between the crystal and PMTs, in which case optimum light transfer is achieved by matching the refractive index of the guide to that of the crystal (Svedberg, 1972). Spatial resolution can be improved by dispensing with the light guide, so bringing the PMTs closer to the scintillation, but this will degrade linearity. Non-linearity can be corrected either electronically or by a variable-density optical mask.

The number of PMTs used will affect both resolution and linearity and the most effective coverage of the crystal is achieved by arranging them in a close-packed hexagonal pattern. Resolution will be best when the photo-cathode area is maximised, but larger photocathodes tend to show non-uniform response across the photo-cathode face with consequent degradation of intrinsic resolution. Large field of view cameras use 37 PMTs with 3-in.-diameter photo-cathodes, although 61 and 91 2-in. tubes are becoming more common. Closer packing of PMTs has been achieved by using an hexagonal photo-cathode.

With the introduction of the more efficient bialkali photo-cathodes in 1967, intrinsic resolution improved by 20–25% (Zimmerman, 1977). Typically, the intrinsic resolution of a large field of view camera is 4 mm at 140 keV. Recent improvements include the use of "tea-cup" photo-cathodes which have a more uniform response across the photo-cathode face, although the actual improvement produced by them is debatable (Perysh and Moi, 1978). A fundamental change in PMT design is probably required to effect a significant improvement in detector system performance.

3.3.3 Pulse arithmetic

The pulse arithmetic circuits are responsible for converting the combined outputs from the PMT array into two signals giving the spatial coordinates of the scintillation, usually denoted as X and Y, and a signal Z indicating the energy of the event.

To achieve this, each PMT has two weighting factors applied to its output signal, one producing its contribution to the X coordinate and the other to the Y value. The final X and Y signals are obtained by summing the signals from all tubes. Thus if W_{xi} is the X weighting factor for the ith tube, then

$$X = \sum_i W_{xi} n_i(x) \tag{3.18}$$

where $n_i(x)$ is the number of photons received by the ith tube when a scintillation occurs at location x. The Y signal is computed in a similar fashion.

The values for the weighting factors will obviously depend upon the shape of $n_i(x)$. The simplest possible case is shown in Fig. 3.13 for a one-dimensional array of nine tubes. In Fig. 3.13b, $n_i(x)$ is shown as triangular with full width at half maximum height equal to the tube separation. To produce a position signal, the sum of the weighted signals should vary linearly with x as in Fig. 3.13d. Conventionally the centre PMT is taken as the origin of the co-ordinate system. Simply summing $n_i(x)$ will give a constant signal as in Fig. 3.13c. This signal is proportional to the energy of the gamma ray, as we are treating the array of PMTs as a single tube. To produce a position signal, then, the weighting factor must be proportional to the x coordinate of the tube's centre, negative weightings for tubes to the left of centre being achieved by subtracting their contribution from the total. For this example,

$$X = 4[n_9(x) - n_1(x)] + 3[n_8(x) - n_2(x)]$$
$$+ 2[n_7(x) - n_3(x)] + [n_6(x) - n_4(x)] \qquad (3.19)$$

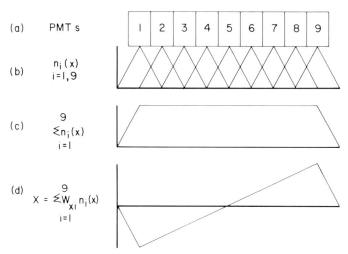

FIG. 3.13. Use of signal weighting to give positional information. (a) A linear array of 9 PMTs. (b) The number of photons $n_i(x)$ received by the $i$thPMT when the scintillation is at position x in the crystal. It is assumed to be a triangular function whose width is equal to the diameter of a PMT. (c) If the PMT signals are simply summed then $\Sigma_i n_i(x)$ is independent of x except at the very edges. This is the signal used to measure the energy Z deposited in the scintillation crystal by the gamma ray. (d) The sum of the weighted signals varies linearly with x.

In practice W_{xi} is a combination of the applied weighting factor k_{xi} and the gain g_i of the tube, i.e.,

$$W_{xi} = k_{xi}g_i \tag{3.20}$$

Figure 3.14 shows a schematic diagram of one of the earliest cameras (Anger, 1958). Position weights k_{xi} and k_{yi} are produced by resistors with values calculated as in the preceding model. For example, tube 3 has an X weighting factor, R_{23}, which is twice that for tube 4, R_{24}, since the X

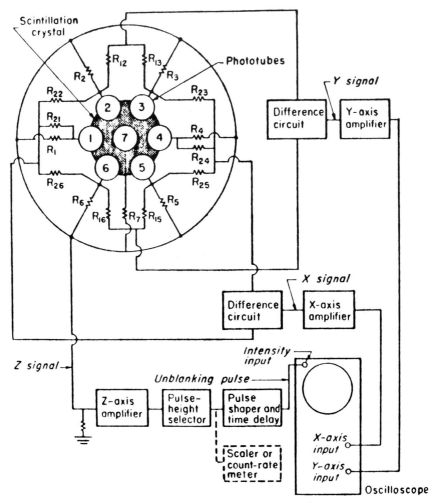

FIG. 3.14. Pulse arithmetic circuit of an early gamma camera. [From Anger (1958).]

coordinate of tube 3 is half that of 4. The difference circuits are used to produce negative weightings; for the X-coordinate calculation the sum of the weighted signals from tubes 2, 1 and 6 is subtracted from that of tubes 3, 4 and 5.

The energy signal Z is computed in the conventional way simply by summing the unweighted output from all the tubes. In Fig. 3.14, the signals are summed through identical resistors $R_1–R_7$.

Since about 30 eV of gamma-ray energy is required to produce one scintillation photon, at low energies the number of photons received by each tube will be small and so have a large statistical variability. In addition the signal from a PMT is affected by changes in quantum efficiency of the photo-cathode, efficiency of collection of electrons at the first dynode, etc. The net result is that the computed energy signal Z produced by photo-electric interactions of a particular gamma emission will vary. The energy resolution of a modern gamma camera (the ratio of the full width at half maximum height of the photo-peak spectrum to the photopeak energy) is about 12%. As can be seen from Eq. (3.19) and (3.20), since in a given camera g_i and k_i are predefined, variations in n_i due to the preceding causes will affect positional computation. Stochastic variations affect intrinsic resolution while non-random changes, such as loss of photons from events near the crystal edge, affect linearity.

Non-random changes can be reduced by employing a narrow window on the pulse height analyser, so reducing the range of values of Z whch produce acceptable signals, but this has the disadvantage of reducing sensitivity. A further limitation of this simple arithmetic is that if a different radionuclide is used, emitting a higher-energy gamma ray, then the average value of n_i will increase and the image becomes larger.

These problems can be reduced by normalising the coordinate signal with the energy signal (Mallard and Myers, 1963). Using this ratio arithmetic the coordinate signal is

$$X = \sum_i k_i g_i n_i(x) \Big/ \sum_i g_i n_i(x) \tag{3.21}$$

Image size thus becomes independent of energy, linearity is improved and although resolution at the crystal centre is not affected, it is improved at the periphery of the field of view.

In practice $n_i(x)$ is not a simple triangular function, a fuller discussion of the calculation of weighting factors can be found in Barrett and Swindell (1981). One consequence of this is that the energy signal may vary with scintillation position, and a set of weighting factors may be necessary to rectify this. Such an energy correction is common in modern cameras. However as Svedberg (1968) has noted, the divisor in the ratio circuit calculation [Eq. (3.21)] should be the unweighted sum of the PMT outputs, not the corrected energy signal.

The pulse arithmetic just described is satisfactory if the only requirement is that the position signal be linearly related to the scintillation position. It takes no account, however, of the need for good spatial resolution which depends upon the noise associated with the PMT signals. Tanaka and colleagues (Tanaka *et al.*, 1970; Hiramoto *et al.*, 1971) considered the problem of computing weighting factors which optimised both linearity and resolution. They found that the contribution k_i that a PMT should make to the final position signal is given by

$$k_i \propto (dn_i(x)/dx)/n_i(x) \qquad (3.22)$$

The weighting factor should be proportional to the fractional rate of change with position of the number of photoelectrons reaching the first dynode. Unfortunately this requires that the value used for the weighting factors is dependent upon the position x of the scintillation. As shown in Fig. 3.15 when the scintillation is directly under tube PM4, n_4 will change very little with small variations in scintillation position, i.e., n_4 contributes little to the calculation of the position signal. However when the scintillation is beneath PM3 or PM5, then n_4 changes rapidly with

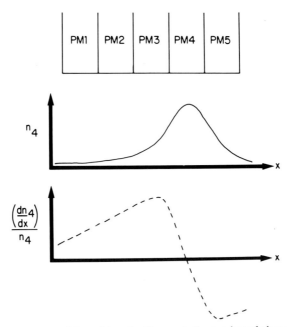

FIG. 3.15. Delay line position arithmetic. Here n_4 is the number of photo-electrons from PMT 4 as a function of the position x of the scintillation. The dashed curve shows the ideal weighting factor k_4.

scintillation position. Thus, the weighting factor should be least for the signal from the PMT nearest to the scintillation but greatest for signals from the neighbouring tubes.

This ideal weighting scheme is achieved in practice by using delay line arithmetic (Tanaka *et al.*, 1970; Hiramoto *et al.*, 1971). The signals from the PMTs are fed into a delay line DL (Fig. 3.16) so that the time of arrival at the end of the line of the pulse from a PMT is proportional to the X or Y coordinate of that tube. The output from the delay line is then clipped by delay lines DL2 and DL3 so that the pulse shape is bipolar symmetrical. By suitable choice of pulse shape, it can be arranged that the zero crossing time of the sum of these pulses is linearly proportional to the X (or Y) coordinate of the event. The time signal is then changed into a conventional voltage position signal by the time-to-pulse height converter. By making the shape of the PMT signals (as a function of time) similar to that of k_i (as a function of distance) position arithmetic close to the ideal model could be achieved. The energy signal Z is produced in the conventional manner by summing the PMT signals. This is used only for pulse height analysis since there is no need to use ratio circuits with this form of pulse arithmetic.

Figure 3.15 also demonstrates that the signals from tubes farthest from the scintillation should be given a low weighting, these signals being of low intensity and so associated with the most noise. In the fixed weighting system, signals from peripheral tubes receive the largest weighting, yet for a scintillation anywhere in the crystal some of these tubes will be most distant from the scintillation.

Kulberg and van Dijk (1972) proposed eliminating these weak signals from the position arithmetic circuits by using a threshold preamplifier in which low-input signals produce no output while higher, and so less noisy, signals are amplified linearly.

3.3.4 Display

The gamma camera display has changed little from that described in Anger's first paper. Voltages proportional to the X and Y co-ordinate signals are applied to the deflection plates of an oscilloscope. If the energy pulse has been passed by the pulse height analyser, then the oscilloscope intensity signal is unblanked, thus causing a spot to appear briefly on the oscilloscope face at a position related to that of the original event in the scintillation crystal. A permanent image is produced by integrating the scintillations on photographic film. For high-quality images the spot size must be kept small and the phosphor response must not vary across the oscilloscope face.

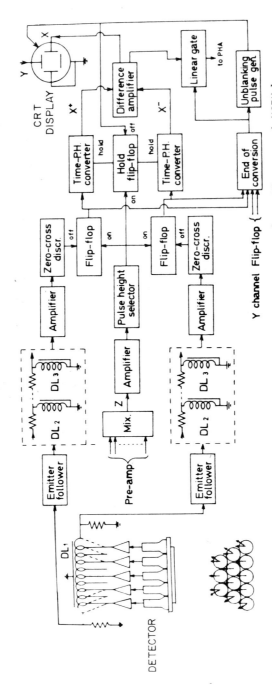

FIG. 3.16. Block diagram of a camera using delay line position arithmetic. [From Hiramoto *et al.* (1971).]

A persistence oscilloscope may also be used to facilitate patient positioning: the long phosphor persistence time provides a degree of integration of the spots to give a recognisable image which is also being continually updated. Such an image is not suitable for recording or analysis.

Multiformatting systems (Section 7.1.1), which allow a far greater flexibility than can be achieved with the simple oscilloscope display, are now becoming standard. Digital displays, using up to a 512×512 element matrix, have been used in place of the analogue display.

3.3.5 Uniformity

When a uniform distribution of activity is imaged on a gamma camera, it will show areas of above- and below-average count density (Fig. 3.17). These non-uniformities are a cause for concern as they may be mistaken for areas of abnormal radiopharmaceutical concentration, so suggesting abnormal pathology (Van Tuinen *et al.*, 1978).

The cause of this non-uniformity can be attributed to variations in the performance of the camera at different points on the detector face, i.e., non-stationarity. More specifically, four causes have been proposed:

(i)   spatial non-linearity
(ii) spatial variation in the energy signal
(iii) spatial variation in detector sensitivity and
(iv) spatial variation in resolution.

Of these factors, (i) and (ii) appear to be the most important (Todd-Pokropek *et al.*, 1976; Wicks and Blau, 1979). For example, a non-linearity of 1 mm in 1 cm may cause a 20% change in count density. Since a single pulse height analyser is used for all energy signals, variations between different PMTs will mean that an interaction in one part of the crystal may produce a signal acceptable to the analyser, while if it occurred at another location in the crystal it would be rejected. While this can be corrected by adjusting the tube gains to give a uniform flood image, the introduction of scattered radiation will cause the image to become non-uniform once again. Variations in detector sensitivity and spatial variations in resolution are said to be small (Todd-Pokropek *et al.*, 1977) and will not be considered further.

A common method of uniformity correction uses the digitised image of a uniform flood source. For each image pixel i, a correction factor $f(i)$ is calculated so that multiplication of the original count density $c(i)$ of this pixel by this factor will adjust the count density to the mean value of the

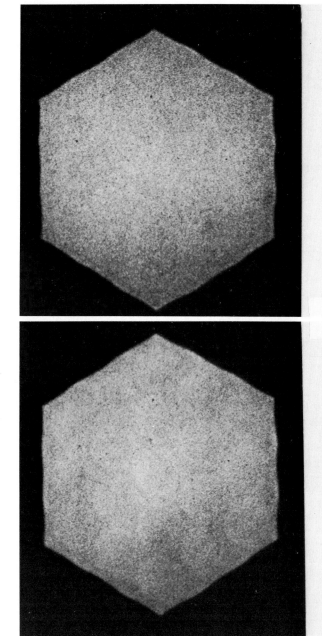

UNCORRECTED   CORRECTED

FIG. 3.17. Image of a uniform flood source of radioactivity before and after uniformity correction.

image *m*, i.e.,

$$f(i) = m/c(i) \tag{3.23}$$

Initially such a correction could only be performed off-line using a data processor and so was limited to digitised images. With the development of micro-processor technology, on-line correction of both analogue and digitised images became possible. As in the off-line method, a flood image is first collected and stored in a memory and correction factors computed according to the degree of non-uniformity. In the circuit shown in Fig. 3.18, each event is temporarily stored in a sample-and-hold circuit. A random number is generated and compared with the correction factor corresponding to the spatial location of the event. If the random number exceeds the value of the correction factor, then the event is displayed, i.e., the unblank signal is allowed. The net effect is to reject counts from hot areas so as to reduce the mean display count density to that of the lowest areas. Figure 3.17 also shows the image after correction. Another form of this on-line correction involves modulating the intensity of the spot on the display scope, usually by varying the length of the unblank signal. Both methods involve discarding counts rather than repositioning them, and although the percentage of rejected counts is low (of the order of 10%), care is required in precise quantitative studies.

These methods for uniformity correction are strictly valid only if variation in detector sensitivity is responsible for non-uniformity. This is now recognised not to be the case, and cameras now incorporate technology to correct for the two main causes, spatial linearity and variations in the energy signal. This circuitry applies position-dependent correction factors to the *X*, *Y* or *Z* signal. For the linearity correction these factors are generated in the factory using special test patterns. A large number of

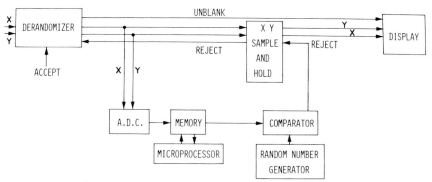

Fig. 3.18. Simplified block diagram of the on-line uniformity correction circuit used in the Technicare Sigma 410 gamma camera.

factors, typically a 1024×1024 array, is necessary as camera uniformity is affected by even small non-linearities.

While spatial non-linearity is mainly dependent upon the design of the camera and so should not alter significantly during the camera's lifetime, energy response may change over a relatively short period owing to deterioration in optical coupling of the tubes to the crystal, ageing of the crystal, etc. It is necessary, therefore, for energy correction factors to be updatable by the operator. This is usually done by acquiring a flood image on the camera. Typically, a 64×64 correction matrix is used.

3.3.6 Performance at high count rates

One of the strengths of the gamma camera is its ability to perform rapid sequential imaging, but reasonable photon densities can only be achieved in such studies by using high photon fluxes. The curve of Fig. 3.19 shows how a gamma camera response might vary with count rate. Initially, the recorded count rate is linearly related to the input count rate, but by about 20 kcps there is a noticeable loss of recorded counts, this deviation from linearity becoming progressively worse. Thus at high count rates there is loss of image contrast, inaccuracy in data quantification and also spatial distortion. As the maximum input count rate encountered in clinical imaging may be as high as 70 kcps, it can be seen that camera performance does not match clinical requirements.

It is important to note that the input count rate shown in Fig. 3.19 refers to those events falling inside the pulse height analyser window, assuming that the camera's response was linear. The actual number of gamma rays

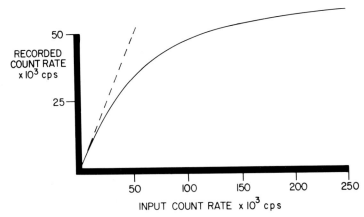

FIG. 3.19. Variation of the count rate recorded by a gamma camera as the true input count rate is increased. The dashed line shows the expected linear response if no count losses occur.

interacting with the crystal and being processed by the electronics prior to pulse height analysis may be three or four times higher than this value.

Data loss and distortion are caused both by the response of the scintillation crystal and by the camera electronics. A scintillation in an NaI(Tl) crystal has a decay time constant of about 0.2 μsec and about 0.8 μsec is required for maximum light collection (Anger, 1958). At high count rates there is an increasing probability that two events will occur within this time and consequently signals will overlap. The camera electronics may see these two (or more) nearly coincident events as one signal, the resulting position and energy being a combination of the individual events. If these so-called pile-up pulses result from low-energy events such as Compton interactions, the recorded energy may fall within the pulse height window, and the event is accepted as real. Spatial distortion thus occurs. Figure 3.20 shows a flood image at low and high count rates; at high count rates the pile-up results in an apparent concentration of events at the crystal centre. The effect of pile-up will depend on the source configuration and the efficiency of the camera electronics. Strand and Larsson (1978) showed that at an expected count rate of 70 kcps, between 5 and 15% of the recorded counts were pile-up. The effect of pile-up is clearly seen in the shape of the energy spectrum which becomes progressively flatter at high count rates.

Crystal response is not the only factor to be considered, the electronic signal processing time also being a major limitation on performance. The signal from the preamplifiers in one camera, for example, has a rapid rise time but a long tail of the order of 50 μsec. Therefore before further handling, the pulses must be shaped, in this case by delay lines which produce a flat top signal of about 1 μsec. As ac coupling of the various amplifiers can result in base-line shifts of the signals with resulting amplitude changes, most cameras now employ base-line restoration circuits.

The shaped signals must pass through summing, weighting and pulse height analyser units before display and in each unit a minimum processing time is required before a new signal can be accepted. Since pulses arriving close to each other are likely to have been distorted, paired-pulse rejection circuits are used in the pulse height analyser circuit to reject both pulses.

Pulse handling can be simplified by derandomizing the signals and storing them in a series of buffers which are then regularly sampled. Since the amount of processing that a signal undergoes affects temporal resolution, some manufacturers offer a high count-rate option facility in which correction circuits, such as those for spatial non-linearity, are bypassed. While image quality will suffer, count-rate losses are reduced significantly.

Since the effect of camera processing time is to distort both positional and energy information, simple mathematical corrections for data loss are

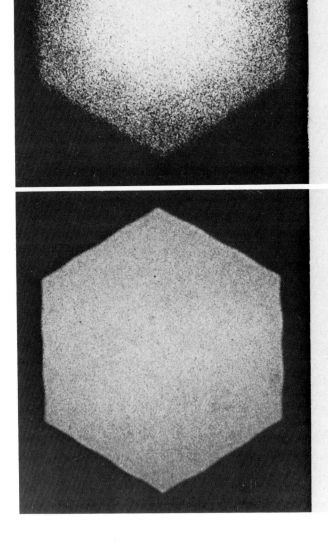

LOW COUNT RATE   HIGH COUNT RATE

FIG. 3.20. Image of a uniform flood source of radioactivity at low and high count rates.

not valid, and for accurate imaging, data rates must be kept within the capabilities of the camera. This problem will be considered further in Chapter 5.

3.3.7 Variations on the standard camera

3.3.7.1 The mobile camera

One of the limitations of radionuclide imaging is that neither the standard gamma camera nor the rectilinear scanner is a portable device. With the increasing importance of cardiac work, the need for a mobile camera which could be used on the ward was evident. One such mobile camera is shown in Fig. 3.21. Like most mobiles, it is designed primarily for cardiac work and so has a small field of view (30 cm) and a 6-mm-thick crystal. On-board data processing systems are also necessary. Performance of these cameras is comparable with that of the standard camera.

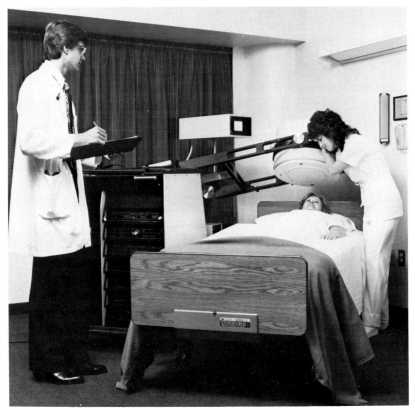

FIG. 3.21. Mobile gamma camera. (Photograph provided by courtesy of International General Electric Medical Systems.)

3.3.7.2 *The scanning camera*

Another limitation of the camera is that whole-body imaging requires seven or eight separate views from both the anterior and posterior aspects. While this does not necessarily inconvenience the patient, the data is not presented in a convenient form for clinical reporting.

In the scanning camera (Fig. 3.22) the detector is moved on rails along the length of the patient, the Y position signals having applied to them an offset which is a function of detector position. Thus, at the completion of the scan a single image is available covering the complete length of the patient (Fig. 3.23). To facilitate imaging, the camera's field of view is usually masked so as to be rectangular. To cover the complete width of the patient, either two scans must be carried out or a diverging 'fish-tail' collimator used (Section 3.3.1.3). While the latter will introduce some distortion into the image, it obviously reduces scanning time by about one half. Figure 3.23 has been produced with such a collimator attached to a camera with a large (50-cm-diameter) field of view.

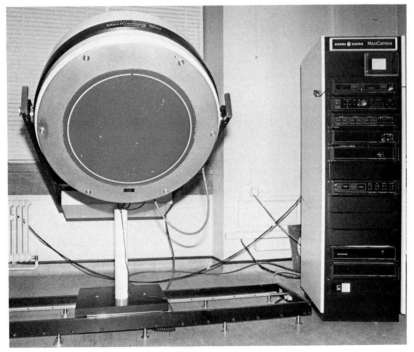

FIG. 3.22. Scanning gamma camera.

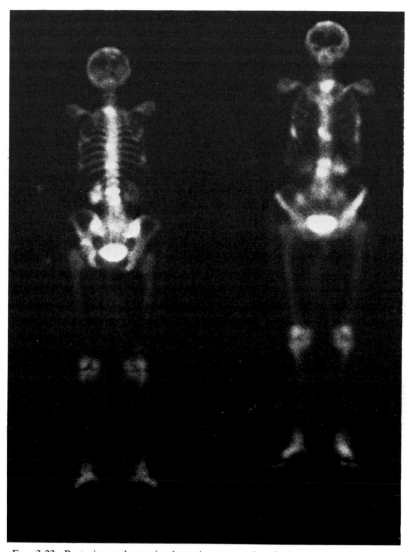

FIG. 3.23. Posterior and anterior bone images produced with a scanning camera.

3.4 Low-resolution imaging with a whole-body counter

3.4.1 Introduction

The philosophy behind the whole-body counter is to produce an instrument that has high sensitivity and accuracy but has little or no imaging capability. Both stationary and scanning whole-body counters have been described in the literature (IAEA, 1970). In the former, neither the patient nor the detector moves, no spatial information is obtained and the prime concern is to measure the lowest possible levels of activity. At the limits of sensitivity, heavy shielding is required and comprises steel, lead or rock that contains a low inherent level of radioactivity. The best whole-body counters can probably detect activities as low as 5 Bq. However, since they have no imaging capabilities, they are outside the scope of this book. For a general review of the subject, the reader is referred to Andrews *et al.* (1973).

The emphasis in this section will be on instruments that, by means of movement either of the detectors or of the patient, provide some information on the distribution of radioactivity in the body, albeit at low resolution. This information may be used in basically two different ways, either to provide data on the absolute percentage of tracer in a given area at a given time, or to provide quantitative data on the turnover of tracer in a particular area of the body during long-term studies.

In recent years whole-body counting has been used primarily in conjunction with neutron activation analysis of selected body constituents, especially calcium (IAEA, 1979). Since neutrons from nuclear reactors are not generally available for medical applications, a number of other sources have been used, including a mixture of americium and beryllium and 252-californium. The latter has a number of advantages (Boddy *et al.*, 1974) including a much smaller volume for the same neutron yield and only about one-fifth the initial cost. Furthermore, the fission spectrum of 252-Cf is of lower energy and consequently easier to moderate. The relatively short half-life of 2.6 yr is unlikely to be a problem in practice because existing sources provide many more neutrons than are normally required for activation work. Deuterium–tritium generators are also capable of producing copious supplies of neutrons for activation analysis by the exothermic fusion reaction

$$^2_1D + {}^3_1H \longrightarrow {}^4_2He + n + 17.6 \text{ MeV}$$

The monoenergetic neutrons must be moderated before use.

When subjects are exposed to a beam of partially moderated fast neutrons, a wide range of reactions are induced; some examples are 48-Ca (n,γ) 49-Ca; 37-Cl (n,γ) 38-Cl; 31-P (n,α) 28-Al and 23-Na (n,γ) 24-Na. All the products emit readily detectable gamma rays when they decay. Since neutron irradiation can be confined to parts of the body, regional information can be obtained by neutron activation analysis. For example, Smith and Tothill (1979) developed apparatus to measure calcium changes in the forearm and spine using 252-Cf. However, in this type of work no imaging capability is required of the detecting system since the region of interest has been defined by the irradiation geometry. Hence, more detailed consideration of this and other applications of neutron activation analysis are outside the scope of this book. [For further reading see IAEA (1979).]

However, a number of problems of calibration, normalisation and reproducibility associated with detection of small temporal changes in body elements are common to all forms of whole-body counting (Kennedy *et al.*, 1982). For example, natural variations in body dimensions, and the difficulty of obtaining a suitable, variable phantom of known composition for calibration mean that absolute quantitation is difficult to achieve. Some of these problems will, therefore, be considered in greater detail.

3.4.2 General problems with whole-body counting

The first problem is that the counter may have to measure a wide range of radionuclides, and hence of gamma-ray energies, and also a very wide range of activities. At the lowest level of activity, ingested radionuclides from the environment such as 137-Cs and 131-I must be measured. Higher up the scale, occupational surveillance of, for example, reactor and fuel processing operators and personnel in biochemistry and nuclear medicine laboratories is important, and ingestion resulting from radiation accidents must be estimated. Many groups have looked at natural 40-K levels (3 Bq/person). This involves no additional radiation burden from adminis-tered activity and has been used for studies during pregnancy. Other medical investigations have used 51-Cr, 57-Co, 58-Co, 60-Co and 75-Se, and recent studies of trace-element metabolism have involved the use of 64-Cu, 67-Cu, 65-Zn and 69m-Zn, amongst others. Measured activities may range from about 5 Bq to 300 kBq.

The greatest sensitivity would be achieved if the patient were totally surrounded by detectors—so-called 4π geometry. However, counting uniformity is increased by placing the detectors some distance away from the patient and arranging them in a predetermined geometric relationship with the body, thus, extremely large detectors would be required. Thus, although a counter with 4π geometry that can measure a few tens of becquerels of a high-energy isotope such as 59-Fe has been reported (Braunsfurth *et al.*, 1977), such an arrangement is scarcely practical for routine hospital work, and even large detector systems (see Smith and Cronquist, 1977) may only collect 10–12% of the available counts.

Liquids, plastics and NaI(Tl) crystals have all been used as scintillation detectors. Liquid scintillators are relatively inexpensive, so large volumes can be used giving good geometric sensitivity. However, there are a number of problems. First a large number of PMTs is required to record the scintillations. Second, since most interactions are Compton processes, energy resolution is inherently poor. Although this may be relatively unimportant when a known radionuclide is being measured, imaging applications require good energy resolution to assist discrimination against scatter. Finally, there are problems with containment, fire and toxicity hazards. Plastic scintillators are more durable, sensitive, stable and of relatively low cost, properties that should make them more attractive for clinical use. However, the NaI(Tl) crystal, the advantages of which were discussed in Section 2.1.3, has been the scintillant of choice for the majority of whole-body counters. The major drawback in this particular context is the high cost of large area detectors.

Most problems arise when whole-body counters are to be used for careful quantitative work. For example, the amount of self attenuation in the patient will vary with the energy of the radiation being detected, the size of the patient and the distribution of radioactivity with depth within the patient. The simplest approximation in correcting for these effects is to assume uniform geometry. This is an easily reproducible condition, and many radionuclides do distribute more or less uniformly in the body. Measurements can be made using different sized phantoms, with variations in both length and equivalent body weight. Note that when a counter is used in the imaging mode, measurements that assume uniform distribution of activity are of limited value since the primary purpose will be to investigate variations in activity from one part of the body to another.

To a first approximation, correction can be made for the depth of activity in the body by combining counts from detectors above and below the patient. Theoretically, for a source of strength I_0 at an arbitary depth Z in a slab of material of thickness l and with linear attenuation coefficient μ, the signal appearing on one side of the slab is

$$I_1 = I_0 e^{-\mu Z} \tag{3.24}$$

and the signal appearing on the other side is

$$I_2 = I_0 e^{-\mu(l-Z)} \tag{3.25}$$

Hence the geometric mean is given by

$$(I_1 I_2)^{1/2} = I_0 e^{-\mu l/2} \tag{3.26}$$

and is independent of Z. In practice, because of scatter, the effective value of μ will not be that for narrow-beam, scatter-free conditions, and Tothill and Galt (1971) have shown that for many X-ray energies the arithmetic mean may be used as an acceptable approximation for calculating the activity.

The expression in Eq. (3.26) depends on the effective patient thickness for gamma-ray attenuation, and this must be estimated. If the density and mean atomic number are approximately constant across the body, attenuation is related to the actual patient thickness, which may be obtained using calipers or a ruler. Otherwise, for example in the thorax, it may be necessary to make gamma-ray transmission measurements using, say, a source of 99m-Tc. The dose to the skin will be quite small, probably less than 10 μGy for 80 MBq of activity. Note that the effective value of μ tends to be somewhat higher for these transmission measurements because the beam is more collimated.

Other errors arise from non-uniformity of the detectors, instability of counter performance, variations in the level of background activity and counting statistics. A fuller discussion of the problems associated with quantification of radionuclide uptake is presented in more general terms in Section 8.2.6.

In many situations it is possible to check the accuracy of calibration factors by making whole-body measurements on patients shortly after administration of a known quantity of radioactivity, i.e., before any excretion has occurred. Some of the problems are less severe if sequential measurements are made on the same patient, although possible redistribution of the activity must be taken into consideration. With care, the whole body activity of a known radionuclide can probably be measured to better than 5%.

3.4.3   One dimensional and two-dimensional imaging

In scanning counters, either the couch or the detectors may move. A design incorporating fixed detectors requires a room approximately twice the patient's length but is otherwise more flexible than one in which the detectors move. For example, in the latter case great care must be taken to shield the PMTs from variations in magnetic fields which could upset the gain and hence energy calibration. Designs with both counters totally enclosed in steel rooms and so-called 'shadow shield' whole-body monitors, in which carefully positioned partial shielding is used [for early designs see Palmer and Roesch (1965) and Boddy (1967)] have been adapted for scanning. If, for example, a shadow shield whole-body monitor is fitted with a single-slit collimator, it may be used for profile scanning which gives one-dimensional information on the distribution of activity in the patient. Several such systems have been constructed. Tothill and Galt

(1971) described a modified whole body counter consisting of two 12.7-cm diameter NaI(Tl) crystals 9 cm thick and 70 cm apart in a 10-cm-thick lead shadow shield. Opposed detectors were used to minimise variation of response with source depth, and each detector was fitted with a single, 10-cm-deep slit collimator with variable separation up to 20 cm. The patient couch speed was variable between 21 and 190 cm min^{-1}.

For a single-slit collimator, resolution is directly proportional to the vertical distance of the source from the crystal and to collimator width. For a detector of constant width, sensitivity is approximately proportional to the square of the collimator opening and to the reciprocal of the source–detector distance. In the latter respect, the system sensitivity is intermediate between a wide-angled fixed detector which follows the inverse square law and a two-dimensional scanning device in which the response to an extended source is independent of the source–detector distance.

Table 3.3 shows typical values of sensitivity and resolution obtained by Tothill and Galt when a point source was scanned using different slit collimator widths. Note the inverse relationship between high sensitivity and good spatial resolution. Comparison with Table 3.2 shows that resolution is much worse than for a gamma camera. However, sensitivity is higher with a detectable limit (accumulated counts approximately equal to background) of about 40 kBq when a point source of 99m-Tc was scanned over a length of 50 cm at 1 cm/sec using a 1-cm collimator slit.

An additional problem with a moving system is that there is a marked fall in counting efficiency when the detector approaches either end of the body (see Fig. 3.24). This is because the detector 'sees' less activity than when it is positioned over the centre of the body. Compensation must be applied, either by using a position-related scaling factor, or by arranging for the scanning speed to be slower when the detector is over the patient's extremities.

TABLE 3.3. Typical values of sensitivity and resolution for a shadow shield whole-body monitor with collimator slits of different widths for 140-keV gamma rays.[a]

Collimator opening (mm)	Sensitivity (counts/photon)	Resolution FWHM (mm)
10	0.8×10^{-4}	31
20	3.4×10^{-4}	62
50	1.9×10^{-3}	148
70	3.5×10^{-3}	200

[a] Scans extended over a length of 50 cm which was sufficient to include the whole profile for the widest collimator considered. The background count rate at 140 keV was 3.0 counts/sec. Adapted from Tothill and Galt (1971).

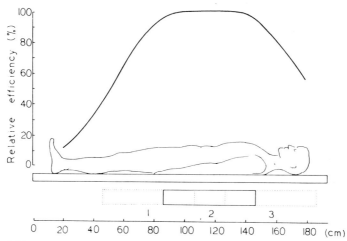

Fig. 3.24. Curve showing how the relative efficiency of a whole-body counter will decrease towards the extremities of the patient. [From Barnaby and Smith (1971).]

There are also problems associated with the interpretation of scans. The first is a direct consequence of poor resolution, which means that the peaks in activity due to separate organs may not be separated. Second, some counts in the image will result from activity in the blood overlying the organ of interest, and a correction must be made for this contribution. The blood-background correction to be applied can be estimated by administering a small quantity of a radiopharmaceutical that will distribute uniformly in the body.

A similar shadow shield whole-body monitor with a slit collimator was used to study copper metabolism in patients, especially in the liver (Walshe and Potter, 1977). When a probe is used for this purpose, there are four major problems. First, the probe must be accurately aligned to "see" the maximum amount of tissue at each viewing, and small variations in positioning result in big variations in recorded count rate. Second, the liver weight must be estimated, and this takes no account of possible liver damage. Third, the thickness of tissue overlying the liver must be estimated to allow for scatter and absorption. Finally it is difficult to obtain information on possible changes in the distribution of copper in other regions of the body at different times and different stages of the disease. All these problems can be partially overcome by developing profile scanning.

Measurements were made using both 67-Cu (half-life = 61.6 h, gamma ray energy = 182 keV) and 64-Cu (half-life = 12.8 h, gamma ray energy = 511 keV). The former is preferable because it can be counted with greater efficiency and for longer but it is much more expensive. The machine was calibrated by recording the response to small sources in known positions, and results are shown in Table 3.4.

Approximately 20 MBq of 64-Cu or 7 MBq of 67-Cu was administered to a patient, and sequential measurements were then made using the profile scanning facility to obtain information on the distribution of activity between the liver and other organs of interest. This work made a significant contribution to showing that the loss of a single gene controlling the handling of copper results in a change in the pattern of uptake by the liver and the efficiency with which the material is cleared by extra-hepatic tissues. Further changes associated with progression of the disease could also be identified.

Two-dimensional scanning gives better positional information but sensitivity is now much lower and the statistical error when attempting to subdivide the signal between different parts of the body is greater. A low-resolution imaging system based on the shadow shield principle has been reported by Gvozdanovic et al. (1981). It consists of four 100-mm-thick × 150-mm-diameter NaI(Tl) crystal detectors arranged two above and two below the patient. Each crystal is fitted with a coarse multi-hole collimator of focal length 300 mm. The detector system is surrounded by 100 mm lead and 20 mm iron to shield against extraneous radiation. The scanning couch is controlled digitally and moves longitudinally through the shadow tunnel, stepping laterally at the end of each passage by a predetermined amount. The spatial resolution (FWHM) at the focal plane is 10 cm for 51-Cr (gamma ray energy = 320 keV) and 12 cm for 59-Fe

TABLE 3.4. Calibration data for a shadow shield whole-body monitor with slit collimator.[a]

Distance of source from couch centre (mm)	Thickness of absorber (mm)	Resolution FWHM (mm)	Relative sensitivity (%)
0	0	69.4	100
75	0	69.4	94
150	0	94.4	88
250	0	150	73
0	23.5	80.6	93
75	23.5	83.3	88
150	23.5	100	80
250	23.5	144	64
0	48.0	88.9	81
0	72.0	94.4	67
0	102	109	52

[a] Adapted from J. M. Walshe and G. Potter, Q. J. Med. **46**, 445–462. Published by Oxford University Press.

(gamma ray energies at 1.10 and 1.29 MeV). A pixel size of 25×25 mm is used to display the data.

With the preceding conditions, the detection limits (a significantly distinguishable image at a scanning speed of 1 pixel/sec) for extended sources of humanoid shape in a supine position are 500 kBq of 51-Cr and 70 kBq of 59-Fe. For a standard format of 16×52 pixels, useful distribution patterns may be obtained from total-body burdens as small as 20 kBq of 65-Zn in scanning times of 30 min.

This scanner has been used to study the metabolism of zinc, which is required in minute quantities as part of many essential co-enzyme systems. If there is a deficiency, keratinisation of the skin, erythema and slow wound healing may result. These are symptoms frequently associated with cirrhosis of the liver. The question to be answered was whether the deficiency resulted from malabsorption of dietary zinc or some other cause.

A dose of 20 kBq of 65-Zn was administered to different groups of patients, and whole-body scans were performed at frequent intervals for many weeks. There was little difference in the observed overall retention of 65-Zn, but when "region of interest" curves were plotted for the liver and skeleton (sacro-iliac region) they showed slow liver clearance and slow bone uptake in normals but much more rapid liver clearance and bone uptake in cirrhotic disease. Hence simple whole-body counting would have shown little difference in total 65-Zn retention for normal and cirrhotic patients, but even with very poor resolution, the scanning technique demonstrates a different pattern of retention. In terms of the clinical problem, this suggests that when zinc is in the liver it is available for incorporation into enzymes, but when it is incorporated into the skeleton (e.g., in cirrhosis) it is irreversibly bound and not available for metabolic incorporation (Gvozdanovic *et al.*, 1982).

Gvozdanovic *et al.* (1985) have improved their data collection and processing procedures to permit simultaneous study of the turn-over of two elements in the body. It is likely that low-resolution high-sensitivity imaging will play an increasing role in studies of the metabolic behaviour of essential trace elements in the future.

3.5 Concluding remarks

In general, the rectilinear scanner has been superseded by the gamma camera primarily because of the need for an imaging device capable of the rapid sequential studies which now form an important part of the work load in a nuclear medicine department. Two points, however, can be made in support of the scanner. First, it is a relatively simple device and can be of great value to departments with limited access to electronic servicing facilities and relatively unreliable power supplies. Second, the rectilinear scanner may be a better imaging device than the camera for higher-energy radionuclides. Not only does the thicker crystal give the scanner a higher sensitivity but the scanner also appears to suffer less from artefacts produced by a high-energy collimator. The septal thickness needed for a high-energy collimator may be such that the septa are resolved by the camera and so produce an intrusive pattern on the image. Alternatively if the septa are made too thin, then excessive penetration produces star-shaped artefacts in the image. These problems do not occur with the rectilinear scanner's focussed collimator.

For most imaging studies, the gamma camera produces images of far better quality than the rectilinear scanner. There may, however, be little further improvement to be made in the spatial resolution of the gamma camera. While changes in detector design may result in further reductions in intrinsic resolution, the collimator resolution cannot be reduced to match it without sacrificing sensitivity.

Until recently, one of the major drawbacks of gamma camera was said to be its non-uniformity. The current generation of cameras, incorporating correction circuits for linearity and energy, give images of very good uniformity and separate flood correction facilities are no longer necessary for routine planar imaging. The temporal resolution is still insufficient for some specialised high-count-rate studies, but gradual replacement of analogue circuitry with digital electronics promises improvements in this direction.

The low-resolution imaging capability of the whole-body counter has, in our opinion, been sadly neglected. Nuclear medicine has, perhaps, been strongly influenced by radiology, and instrument development has largely been aimed at producing high-quality images. The range of radio-pharmaceuticals produced has been constrained by the need for relatively high levels of activity to be used in order to give an image with high count density. Consequently, the value of a device which gives poor quality images but allows the distribution of very small quantities of radioactive materials to be quantitatively measured with high accuracy is not appreci-ated. It is to be hoped that this topic will receive more attention in the future.

References

Andrews, G. A., Gibbs, W. D., Morris. A. C., Jr. and Ross, D. A. (1973). Whole body counting. *Semin. Nucl. Med.* **3,** 367–388.
Anger, H. O. (1958). Scintillation camera. *Rev. Sci. Instrum.* **29,** 27–33.

Anger, H. O. (1964). Scintillation camera with multichannel collimators. *J. Nucl. Med.* **5,** 515–531.

Anger, H. O. and Davis, D. H. (1964). Gamma ray detection efficiency and image resolution in sodium iodide. *Rev. Sci. Instrum.* **35,** 693–697.

Atkins, F. B., Beck, R. N., Hoffer, P. B. and Palmer, D. (1976). Dependence of optimum baseline setting on scatter fraction and detector response function. *In* "Medical Radionuclide Imaging", Vol. 1, pp. 101–118. IAEA, Vienna.

Baker, R. G. and Scrimger, J. W. (1967). An investigation of the parameters in scintillation camera design. *Phys. Med. Biol.* **12,** 51–63.

Barnaby, C. F. and Smith, T. (1971). Calibration of a whole body counter suitable for use in routine clinical investigations. *Phys. Med. Biol.* **16,** 97–104.

Barrett, H. H. and Swindell, W. (1981), "Radiological Imaging. The Theory of Image Formation, Detection and Processing", Vol. 1, pp. 262–268. Academic Press, New York and London.

Beck, R. N. (1964). Collimators for radioisotope scanning systems. *In* "Medical Radioisotope Scanning", pp. 211–231. IAEA, Vienna.

Boddy, K. (1967). A high sensitivity shadow shield whole body monitor with scanning bed and tilting chair geometries, incorporated in a mobile laboratory. *Br. J. Radiol.* **40,** 631–637.

Boddy, K., Robertson, I. and Glaros, D. (1974). The development of a facility for partial body *in-vivo* activation analysis using californium 252 neutron sources. *Phys. Med. Biol.* **19,** 858–861.

Braunsfurth, J. A., Gabbe, E. E. and Heinrich, H. C. (1977). Performance parameters of the Hamburg 4π whole body radioactivity detector. *Phys. Med. Biol.* **22,** 1–17.

Cassen, B., Curtis, L., Reid, C. and Libby, R. (1951). 131I use in medical studies. *Nucleonics* **9,** 46–50.

Ehrhardt, J. C. (1974). Effect of a scattering medium on gamma ray imaging. *J. Nucl. Med.* **15,** 943–948.

Gvozdanovic, D., Ettinger, K. V., Smith, D. B., Taylor, G. G., Gvozdanovic, S. and Mallard, J. R. (1981). Investigations of long term *in-vivo* tracer distribution patterns using an ultra high sensitivity scanning system. *In* "Medical Radionuclide Imaging", Vol. 1, pp. 83–105. IAEA, Vienna.

Gvozdanovic, D., Gvozdanovic, S., Crofton, W. W., Aggett, P. J., Mowat, N. A. G., Brunt, P. W. and Mallard, J. R. (1982). Ultra high sensitivity imaging in study of long term distribution of Zn–65 tracer. *Proc. World Congr. Med. Phys. Biomed. Eng.*, *Hamburg* Abstr. 21–26.

Gvozdanovic, D., Gvozdanovic, S. and Mallard, J. R. (1985). Simultaneous study of two element turnover in human body and organs by radionuclide ultra high sensitivity imaging. *Nutrition Res.* Suppl. 1, 44–47.

Hiramoto, T., Tanaka, E. and Nohara, N. (1971). A scintillation camera based on delay-line time conversion. *J. Nucl. Med.* **12,** 160–165.

IAEA (1970). "Directory of Whole Body Radioactivity Monitors", Data Sheet UK9 1. IAEA, Vienna.

IAEA (1979). "Neutron Activation Techniques in the Life Sciences 1978", STI/PUB/492. IAEA, Vienna.

Kennedy, N. S. J., Eastell, R., Ferrington, C. M., Simpson, J. D., Smith, M. A., Strong, J. A. and Tothill, P. (1982). Total body neutron activation analysis of calcium-calibration and normalisation. *Phys. Med. Biol.* **27,** 697–707.

Kuhl, D. E., Chamberlain, R. H., Hale, J. and Gorson, R. O. (1962). A high contrast photographic recorder for scintillation counter scanning. *Radiology* **66,** 730–739.

Kulberg, G. H. and van Dijk, N. (1972). Improved resolution of the Anger scintillation camera through the use of threshold preamplifiers. *J. Nucl. Med.* **13**, 169–171.

Lakshmanan, A. V., Causer, D. A., Wilks, R. J., Taylor, C. G. and Mallard, J. R. (1975). A "depth-independent" collimator for use with ^{99m}Tc in both conventional and transverse section scanning. *Int. J. Nucl. Med. Biol.* **2**, 123–128.

MacIntyre, W. A., Fedoruk, S. O., Harris, C. C., Khul, D. E. and Mallard, J. R. (1969). Sensitivity and resolution in radioisotope scanning. *In* "Medical Radioisotope Scintigraphy", Vol. 1, pp. 391–434. IAEA, Vienna.

Mallard, J. R. and Myers, M. J. (1963). The performance of a gamma-camera for the visualisation of radioactive isotopes *in-vivo. Phys. Med. Biol.* **8**, 165–182. .

Mallard, J. R. and Peachey, C. J. (1959). A quantitative automatic body scanner for localisation of radioisotopes *in-vivo. Br. J. Radiol.* **32**, 652–659.

Mather, R. L. (1957). Gamma ray collimator penetration and scattering effects. *J. Appl. Phys.* **28**, 1200–1207.

Mayneord, W. V., Turner, R. C., Newbery, S. P. and Hodt, H. J. (1951). A new method for making visible the distribution of activity in a source of ionizing radiation. *Nature (London)* **168**, 762–765.

Moyer, R. A. (1974). A low energy multi-hole converging collimator compared with a pinhole collimator. *J. Nucl. Med.* **15**, 59–64.

Muehllehner, G. (1969). A diverging collimator for gamma ray imaging cameras. *J. Nucl. Med.* **10**, 197–201.

Muehllehner, G., Dudek, J. and Moyer, R. (1976). Influence of hole shape on collimator performance. *Phys. Med. Biol.* **21**, 242–250.

Palmer, H. E. and Roesch, W. C. (1965). A shadow shield whole body counter. *Health Phys.* **11**, 1213–1219.

Perysh, D. E. and Moi, T. E. (1978). State of the art photomultiplier tubes for Anger cameras. *IEEE Trans. Nucl. Sci.* **NS–25**, 615–619.

Royal, H. D., Brown, P. H. and Claunch, B. C. (1979). Effects of a reduction in crystal thickness on Anger camera performance. *J. Nucl. Med.* **20**, 977–980.

Smith, M. A. and Tothill, P. (1979). Development of apparatus to measure calcium changes in the forearm and spine by neutron activation analysis using Californium 252. *Phys. Med. Biol.* **24**, 319–329.

Smith, T. and Cronquist, A. G. (1977). A versatile and economic whole body counter based on liquid scintillation detector modules. *Br. J. Radiol.* **50**, 332–339.

Strand, S. E. and Larsson, I. (1978). Image artifacts at high photon fluence rates in single-crystal NaI (Tl) scintillation cameras. *J. Nucl. Med.* **19**, 407–413.

Svedberg, J. D. (1968). Image quality of a gamma camera system. *Phys. Med. Biol.* **13**, 597–610.

Svedberg, J. D. (1972). On the intrinsic resolution of a gamma camera system. *Phys. Med. Biol.* **17**, 514–524.

Tanaka, E., Hiramoto, T. and Nohara, N. (1970). Scintillation cameras based on new position arithmetic. *J. Nucl. Med.* **11**, 542–547.

Todd-Pokropek, A. E., Erbsmann, F. and Soussaline, F. (1977). The non-uniformity of imaging devices and its impact in quantitative studies. *In* "Medical Radionuclide Imaging", Vol. 1, pp. 67–82. IAEA, Vienna.

Tothill, P. and Galt, J. M. (1971). Quantitative profile scanning for the measurement of organ radioactivity. *Phys. Med. Biol.* **16**, 625–634.

Tyson, R. K. and Amtey, S. R. (1978). Practical considerations in gamma-camera line spread function measurement. *Med. Phys.* **5**, 480–484.

Van Tuinen, R. J., Kruger, J. B., Bahr, G. K. and Sodd, V. J. (1978). Scintillation camera non-uniformity: effects on cold lesion detectability. *Int. J. Nucl. Med. Biol.* **5**, 135–140.

Walshe, J. M. and Potter, G. (1977). The pattern of the whole body distribution of radioactive copper (Cu 67, Cu 64) in Wilson's disease and various control groups. *Q. J. Med.* **46,** 445–462.

Wicks, R. and Blau, M. (1979). Effect of spatial distortion on Anger camera uniformity correction. *J. Nucl. Med.* **20,** 252–254.

Zimmerman, R. E. (1977). Advances in nuclear medicine imaging instrumentation. *In* "Medical Radionuclide Imaging", Vol. 1, pp. 121–139. IAEA, Vienna.

Chapter 4

Tomography

4.1 Introduction

The term tomography has been applied to techniques aimed at visualising one layer or section of the body, in this instance the distribution of radionuclide in that section. Two techniques have evolved and for convenience these are termed "longitudinal" and "transverse" tomography. In longitudinal tomography details in one chosen plane are kept in focus whilst attempts are made to blur detail from all other planes (but inevitably these are still superimposed on the image of the in-focus plane). In transverse tomography information is collected from a single plane at many different angles and an image is reconstructed from this information using mathematical techniques implemented by digital computer.

The conventional radionuclide image represents a projection of the radionuclide concentration in an object onto a plane (Fig. 4.1). The interpretation of the image is an attempt to reconstruct the spatial distribution from the projection. Depth information can be obtained from an orthogonal projection (antero-posterior and lateral being the usual combination), assuming the geometrical relationships which exist amongst points, lines and surfaces in space. However, particularly when dealing with a distribution which varies continuously throughout a volume, this can lead to ambiguity, so the methods of pure solid geometry are insufficient. A series of projections is necessary to infer unambiguously the structure or distribution within the object. The imperfect spatial resolving capabilities of gamma-ray imaging systems invariably lead to a continuously varying

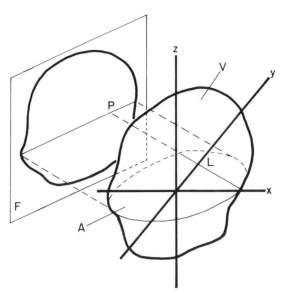

FIG. 4.1. Object and its projection onto a plane.

spatial distribution even though the actual object may have well-defined geometrical detail. If the distribution of radionuclide within a single section can be reconstructed, then since a volume is composed of a series of such sections, we have a complete quantitative solution to the three-dimensional problem, and the radionuclide concentration can be measured at all points within the object.

Figure 4.2 illustrates how a potential contrast of 6 : 1 is reduced to 2 : 1 in a simplified projection scheme. Although an over-simplification, it demonstrates the drawback in "conventional" imaging. The purpose of tomography is to recover this contrast, to determine the true quantitative picture, and if possible even to portray information not perceptible on the conventional views.

4.2 Longitudinal tomography

The first attempts to separate discrete planes were made through the technique of longitudinal tomography, where detail in all planes except one "in-focus" plane is blurred. The simplest method is to use a sharply focussed detection system, e.g., a large crystal scanning detector with short-focus collimator. Objects in the focal plane will then be sharply resolved while objects at all other depths, above and below the focal plane, are poorly resolved with resolution decreasing progressively away from the

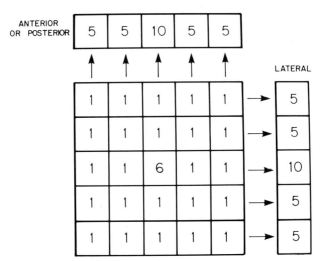

Fig. 4.2. How a potential contrast of 6:1 in the object becomes a contrast of 2:1 in conventional imaging.

focal plane. The detection system is extremely sensitive to objects in the focal plane on account of the large solid angle subtended, but unfortunately it is necessary to preselect the depth of interest within the patient and to carry out a separate study for each selected depth.

However, it was shown by Anger (1969) that if the position of each scintillation occurring within the crystal is also known, then by subtle optical manipulation of the data, several images can be obtained simultaneously, each displaying a different plane in focus with all other planes out of focus. The principle of the Anger tomographic scanning camera is illustrated in Fig. 4.3. [For an assessment of the physical properties of a commercial system see Zenari *et al.* (1983).]

In the upper part of the figure, the three point sources are shown to be in planes *A*, *C* and *E*. As the camera is scanned over the sources (middle) the images of the three sources appear at different positions on the display as shown in the lower part of the figure.

To reconstruct plane *C*, the focal plane of the collimator, no data manipulation is needed and the total camera count rate is attributed to the instantaneous position of the camera as in conventional rectilinear scanning. To reconstruct the activity distribution of other planes, the data in each cathode ray tube (CRT) image is shifted by an amount which depends upon both the position of the camera at that instant and the depth of the desired reconstruction plane. When all the CRT images are summed to give the final image, scintillations resulting from the plane of interest will

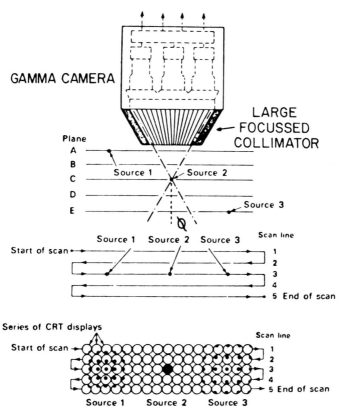

GAMMA CAMERA

LARGE
FOCUSSED
COLLIMATOR

Plane
A
B
C
D
E

Source 1   Source 2

Source 3

Q

Source 1   Source 2   Source 3   Scan line

Start of scan   1
2
3
4
5 End of scan

Series of CRT displays   Scan line

Start of scan   1
2
3
4
5 End of scan

Source 1   Source 2   Source 3

FIG. 4.3. Tomographic scanning gamma camera. Three radioactive point sources on different planes produce very different scintillation patterns over the camera crystal as the scan progresses. By suitable manipulation several images can be produced, each displaying a particular plane in focus. The tomographic effect depends upon the collimator angle ϕ. [From Anger (1969).]

reinforce each other while those from other planes will simply produce a blurred background. This reconstruction process can be carried out either electronically or optically.

Attempts to eliminate the rectilinear scanning motion resulted in the tomographic scintillation camera. This instrument was basically a stationary Anger camera equipped with a parallel slanted-hole collimator and a patient couch with a movable top (Meuhllehner, 1971). The collimator rotates in its housing and at the same time the table top moves in a circular pattern at the same rate of rotation (Fig. 4.4). Again by suitable manipulation of the camera scintillations, several images can be obtained simultaneously, each displaying a different plane in focus. The image of a point

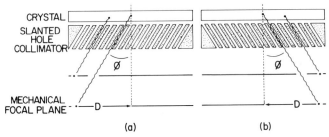

F<small>IG</small>. 4.4. The tomographic scintillation camera—a gamma camera with slanted parallel hole collimator equipped to rotate through 360°. (a) Starting position and (b) after rotation through 180°. If the couch top also rotates in synchronism with the collimator, with radius of rotation D, then only one plane in the object remains in focus (the mechanical focal plane). By suitable manipulation of the scintillations, images of other planes can be simultaneously brought into focus.

source lying above or below the plane of interest will take the form of a doughnut rather than the broad gaussian profile obtained with the Anger tomographic scanning camera, since only one specific value of ϕ is used instead of the whole range of angles from 0 to ϕ. The minimum exposure time is determined by the rate of rotation of the collimator and couch, typically 30 sec/revolution, considerably shorter than the time required to cover the area in a rectilinear raster.

A further development of longitudinal gamma camera tomography is the multiple pinhole approach, which appears useful for relatively small organs, particularly the heart, where rapid serial imaging is often required (Vogel *et al.*, 1978). A pinhole collimator with an array of seven pinholes is used to project seven separate images onto the camera crystal. Each view is at a slightly different angle, a central view with $\phi = 0$, plus six discrete views equally spaced around the central view with ϕ approximately 27°. Digital manipulation of the data can then produce multiple images, each displaying a different longitudinal plane in focus.

Note that for all these instruments the tomographic effect depends essentially on the maximum angle ϕ at which the detector sees the object, and this is generally greater with the tomographic scanning camera. It can be seen that the in-focus plane is not effectively isolated from neighbouring planes.

4.3 Transverse tomography

The technique of transverse radionuclide tomography was proposed by Kuhl and Edwards (1963). It can be considered the limiting form of

longitudinal tomography with $\phi = 90°$. A transverse section of the body
is scanned using a pair of opposed detectors, a single traverse being
obtained at each of a series of angles around the section of interest
(Fig. 4.5). A gamma camera rotating around the patient can also be used
to obtain such a series of angularly spaced profiles. In their original
proposals, Kuhl and Edwards considered a simple optical processing
technique in order to reconstruct an image of the radionuclide distribution
within the section. A CRT display was used and, in a manner similar to
that demonstrated in Fig. 4.5, a line was generated for each position of the
detectors, the intensity of the line on the CRT being proportional to the
combined counting rates from the detectors. The lines were superimposed,
through a time exposure, onto photographic film, and after all the scan
lines had been completed the exposure was terminated and the film
developed.

The method yields an approximation to the actual object distribution in
that peaks and troughs will be reproduced in the correct positions. Such
processing is now accomplished digitally and has come to be known as
"back-projection and superposition of profiles". The same reconstruction
problem arose in a number of specialist sciences, chiefly radioastronomy,
electron microscopy and radiology, and practical solutions to the problem
have been devised, particularly over the last decade, with the help of
digital computing (see, e.g., Smith *et al.*, 1973).

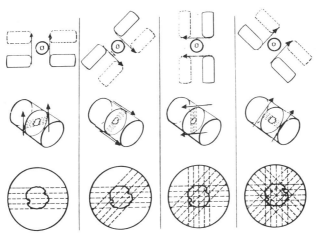

Fɪɢ. 4.5. Transverse section scanning. Activity profiles of the object are obtained at a
series of angles around the section of interest. [From Kuhl (1964).]

4.4   Reconstruction techniques

4.4.1   The problem

Figure 4.6 illustrates more precisely what is meant by a "projection", essentially a line integral of a two-dimensional function $g(x, y)$, in this instance the amount of radioactivity per unit area. In practice, the plane of $g(x, y)$ will be of finite thickness in the z dimension but it is assumed that the function remains fairly constant over this thickness and that $g(x, y)$ is the average value. The area A projects into a line profile on the detection plane, the value of the projected density at P being the line integral of $g(x, y)$ along the straight line L through the object, i.e.,

$$P_\theta(x') = \int g(x, y) \, dy' \tag{4.1}$$

The subscript θ refers to the angle at which the profile is taken; x' and y' are the customary Cartesian co-ordinates in the rotated-system where

$$x' = x \cos \theta + y \sin \theta \tag{4.2}$$

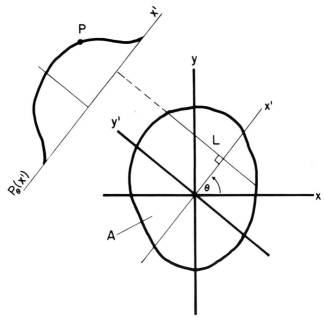

FIG. 4.6. Area A in the x, y plane and its projected profile at angle θ (cf. Fig. 4.1).

The problem is to determine or reconstruct the function $g(x, y)$ over the plane A from a series of profiles $P_\theta(x')$ which are equally spaced in angle θ. A mathematical solution to this theoretical problem was expounded by Radon in 1917 (see Cormack, 1973). Note that the plane A (the section) is truly isolated, free from interference from all other planes, and thus in practice the thickness of the section will depend only on the collimation properties in the z direction. It is assumed that observable data can be related to the true line integrals $P_\theta(x')$; this relationship will be investigated later. Note that the integral of any one profile yields the total radioactivity T within the slice, i.e.,

$$\int P_\theta(x')dx' = \iint g(x,y)\,dx\,dy = T \qquad (4.3)$$

4.4.2 Back-projection

Given a series of N profiles equally spaced at angles π/N, then formally

$$\theta = i\pi/N \qquad i = 0,1, 2, \ldots N - 1$$

and the approximate solution given by simple back-projection is

$$g_1(x,y) = \sum_{\theta=0}^{\pi(1-1/N)} P_\theta(x') \qquad (4.4)$$

where x' is given by Eq. (4.2), i.e., the reconstructed density at a point is assumed to be given by the addition of all projections through that point, and $g_1(x, y)$ is an approximation to $g(x, y)$. Each value of θ specifies one profile, and the value of x' specifies that projection through the point x, y under consideration. As long as $g(x,y)$ has a highly peaked structure, these peaks will appear in the reconstruction; so the method may be said to give an approximate solution. A high background is inevitably obtained, and points outside the object, i.e., where $g(x,y)$ is zero, will have substantially non-zero values in $g_1(x,y)$. A background constant may be subtracted and $(N - 1)T$ has been suggested as a suitable value (Vainstein, 1970) where T is the total radioactivity as defined in Eq. (4.3).

To gain some insight into the effect of this reconstruction process, the impulse response of back-projection may be examined. If the input data corresponding to a single point is considered, each profile consists of a delta function which will back-project into a line, with a resulting image consisting of superimposed lines, as illustrated in Fig. 4.7. The impulse response, therefore, is spatially varying and depends on the number of profiles. For the special case of an infinite number of profiles, the image

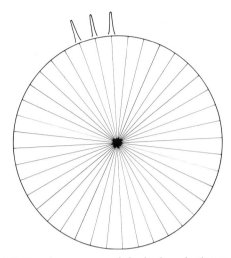

F$_{IG}$. 4.7. Impulse response of the back-projection process.

density, i.e., the limiting value of the line density, is inversely proportional to the radial distance r from the point under consideration. Thus, it is shown that with a sufficient number of profiles the back-projected image in fact represents a convolution of the true image with a known function, which tends to the form $1/r$ in the limiting case of an infinite number of profiles

$$g_1(x,y) = g(x,y) * (1/r)$$

Therefore, it is not unreasonable to expect that we may obtain a better estimate of $g(x,y)$ than that provided by back-projection alone by using the technique of deconvolution. Without being rigorous the rationale is briefly as follows. The Fourier transform of $(1/r)$ is $(1/R)$ where r represents distance in real space and R represents distance in Fourier transform space, also called frequency space or reciprocal space (Smith *et al.*, 1973). The transform of the back-projected image $g_1(x, y)$ therefore represents the transform of the true image multiplied by this $(1/R)$ function, i.e.,

$$T\langle g_1(x,y)\rangle = T\langle g(x,y)\rangle \cdot T\langle 1/r\rangle$$
$$= T\langle g(x,y)\rangle \cdot 1/R$$

Multiplication by R followed by the inverse transform back to real space should yield the true image $g(x,y)$

$$R \cdot T\langle g_1(x,y)\rangle = T\langle g(x,y)\rangle$$
$$T^{-1}[R \cdot T\langle g_1(x,y)\rangle] = g(x,y)$$

An alternative to multiplication in reciprocal space is convolution in real space, using a function whose Fourier transform is R, the ramp function

$$T^{-1}\langle R \rangle * g_1(x, y) = g(x, y)$$

Since back-projection is a linear operation, the convolution may be performed on the raw data projections before the back-projection operation, with the simple advantage of applying the convolution in one-dimensional space. These filtered projections may then be back-projected to form the final image—the technique commonly referred to as filtered back-projection, i.e., the profiles are first filtered to form a new series of projections $H_\theta(x')$ where

$$H_\theta(x') = P_\theta(x') * f(x')$$

and the solution given by filtered back-projection is

$$g_2(x, y) = \sum_{\theta=0}^{\pi(1-1/N)} H_\theta(x') \tag{4.5}$$

a hopefully better approximation to $g(x, y)$.

The form of the filter function f is such that spatial frequencies are amplified, with amplification directly proportional to frequency up to a certain value and thereafter smoothly suppressed to zero at some maximum spatial frequency R_m (Chesler and Riederer, 1975). A typical example is shown in Fig. 4.8. The high-frequency limitation is necessary because of sampling and noise effects in any real data and is also an essential requirement if a finite number of profiles are to suffice. For example, it can be shown that if $g(x, y)$ is a smoothly varying function, containing no spatial frequencies in excess of R_m, then the reconstruction is free of angular sampling artefacts provided that

$$N > \pi R_m D \tag{4.6}$$

where N is the number of profiles and D is the maximum dimension across $g(x, y)$ (Bracewell and Riddle, 1967). By using the filter function shown in Fig. 4.8, N can be reduced below the rather strict limit imposed by Eq. (4.6). Thus, for a given resolution and a given diameter of object, the minimum number of profiles may be specified. For example, a resolution index of 1 cm implies that $R_m = 0.8$ cm^{-1}, approximately, and with a 20-cm-diameter object, strict interpretation of Eq. (4.6) leads to $N > 16\pi$, i.e., about 50 profiles. In practice, given a limitation on the data collection time, 30 profiles at 6° angular increments are generally found to be adequate. If more profiles are attempted, then time per profile must be decreased with resulting poorer counting statistics in each profile and no net improvement. If fewer profiles are attempted, the volume of data is minimised and statistics within each profile may be improved, but the spatial variance of the impulse response of the back-projection process, as illustrated in Fig. 4.7, becomes appreciable with resulting artefacts. By using filters such as illustrated in Fig. 4.8, a practical compromise would appear to be given by

$$N = 2 R_m D$$

4.4.3   Implementation of reconstruction theory

The reconstruction method assumes projections $P_\theta(x')$ corresponding to the line integrals of $g(x, y)$ as in Eq. (4.1). We must now consider how actual data can be related to these line integrals.

For an idealised detection system (as in Chapter 2), whose count rate from point to point is a measure of the flux of gamma rays emitted perpendicular to the detector surface, the response to a source distributed within an attenuating medium is

$$F_\theta(x') \propto \int g(x', y') \exp(-\mu y') \, dy' \, \Delta z \qquad (4.7)$$

where Δz is the thickness of the section, $g(x, y)$ the average value of the radioactivity concentration within the section at location x, y, and

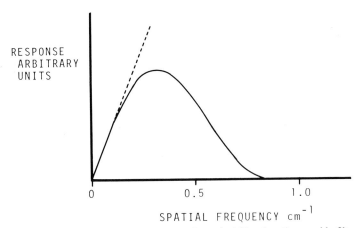

FIG. 4.8. Spatial frequency response curve of a typical filter function used in filtered back projection. The cut-off frequency, 0.8 cm^{-1}, was chosen with due regard to the spatial resolution of the particular imaging device (FWHM = 1 cm approximately)and the statistical accuracy of the measurements (up to 256 counts/measurement).

$\exp(-\mu y')$ represents attenuation in the y' direction (i.e., y' would need to be measured from the surface of the attenuating medium nearest the detector). This is the problem of self-attenuation. The data $F_\theta(x')$ need to be corrected (multiplied by a factor to allow for attenuation) to derive data which approximates to line integrals as required by Eq. (4.1), the starting point of the reconstruction theory.

Furthermore, with practical gamma-ray detection systems the point spread function (PSF) introduces another source of variation within the line integral: a solid angle factor. If $P(x, y, z)$ represents the PSF, then we have already seen (Chapter 2) that observable data are of the form (with suitable adjustment of axes to suit our present considerations)

$$F_\theta(x', z') \propto \int \int \int g(x, y', z) P(x - x', y', z - z') \, dx dz \exp(-\mu y') \, dy' \quad (4.8)$$

where integration is carried out over the entire active volume. The combination of solid angle and attenuation factors within the integral is a major problem in emission tomography, and the consequence is quantitatively inexact reconstructions. However, with all its imperfections, emission tomography has had some success in clinical practice and interest continues, especially with the new generation of rotating gamma cameras and positron imagers. We shall analyse the problems again with the gamma camera particularly in mind.

4.4.3.1 The self-attenuation problem

The extent of self-attenuation can be appreciated from Eq. (4.7), ignoring the solid angle factor for the moment. If $g(x, y)$ represents a uniformly distributed activity within a circle (e.g., a transverse section through a cylinder), then Fig. 4.9 shows the difference between true line integrals, where $\mu = 0$, and those obtained with $\mu = 0.123 \text{ cm}^{-1}$ (an effective attenuation coefficient for 140-keV gamma-rays in water). The true line integral is simply proportional to the chord length L whereas the self-attenuated line integral is proportional to $[1 - \exp(-\mu L)]/\mu$ as was found in Eq. (2.2). The required correction factor for the self-attenuated line integral is simply $\mu L/[1 - \exp(-\mu L)]$, shown in Fig. 4.10. But the correction factor depends on the distribution of radioactivity. For any thickness L, the extreme variations will be given by a source concentrated at the near surface, when self attenuation will be negligible (correction factor 1.0) and a source concentrated at the far surface, when attenuation will be maximum [correction factor $\exp(\mu L)$]. The uniform distribution correction factor lies between these two extremes (Fig. 4.10). In practice the projection is usually measured from the opposite direction as well and

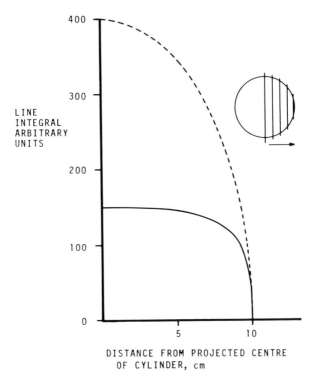

FIG. 4.9. Projected profile of a 20-cm-diameter cylinder. The true line integrals (----) are proportional to the chord length L. The self-attenuated line integrals (——) show the extent of the problem ($\mu = 0.123$ cm^{-1}).

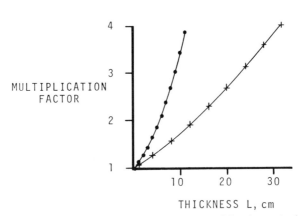

FIG. 4.10. Correction factors for restoring self-attenuated line integrals, for a uniformly distributed source of thickness L (+) and for a source concentrated at depth L from the detector (●). [From Keyes (1979). Copyright © 1979 IEEE.]

the combination of these measurements can considerably reduce the problem. If opposed detector measurements are represented by A and B, then

$$(A + B)\mu L/[1 - \exp(-\mu L)] \simeq \int g(x', y')\, dy' \qquad (4.9)$$

The additional information required, i.e., the thickness of the object for each projection, is considerable. Again a further practical compromise would be to represent a patient section by a defined geometrical shape, for example, an ellipse of homogeneous material. Two dimensions, the major and minor axes, are then sufficient to specify the thickness for each projection (Fig. 4.11) (Keyes, 1976).

A further complication occurs in practice if μ varies appreciably throughout the medium, i.e., if the tissues containing the radionuclide are of different densities. Further approximations are then called for, and iterative procedures would seem to be required, provided the initial data is sufficiently accurate to warrant lengthy computation (Rowe, 1979; Gullberg, 1979)

4.4.3.2 The solid angle problem

Returning to Eq. (4.8), we can investigate the effect of the solid angle factor, i.e., the inclusion of the PSF within the line integral. By using

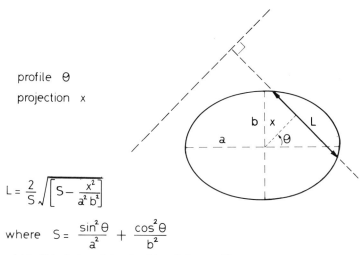

FIG. 4.11. Calculation of the chord length for an ellipse. Two measurements, the major and minor axes, are sufficient to specify the thickness L for any projection at distance x from the centre of the ellipse. [From Keyes (1976).]

experiments with line sources suspended in air, the effect of attenuation can be excluded in order to study the effect of solid angle alone (Rowe and Keyes, 1979). Figure 4.12 shows the experimental arrangement. Because of the averaging effect of the data collection process (the detector obtains views at many different angles with different distances between source and detector in each view), the reconstructed peak value of a line source in air is surprisingly constant, independent of its radial distance from the centre of rotation (Fig. 4.13). This was found to be true for both a rotating gamma camera system and a focussed collimator scanning system, i.e., systems with quite different PSFs.

When an attenuating medium is present and a reconstruction is performed without any attenuation correction, then the reconstructed peak values demonstrate considerable position dependence—a factor of more than 2 between central and peripheral positions. Figure 4.13 thus becomes a calibration curve to enable measurement of the line source activity from the reconstructed peak value, specifically for this one set of conditions (diameter of material D, separation S, energy window, etc.). For point sources of activity, a slightly different calibration would be obtained due to the different variation of point and line spread functions with distance from the detector.

Thus, realistic reconstructions are possible given a detection system with reasonably parallel geometry. Attenuation correction is of the utmost

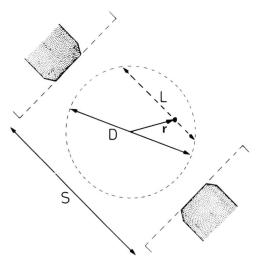

FIG. 4.12. Experimental arrangement for studying a line source at a radial distance r from the centre of rotation of the scanner or camera detection system. The line source is placed inside a cylinder, of diameter D of attenuating material. Here S is the separation. [From Rowe and Keyes (1979). Copyright © 1979 IEEE.]

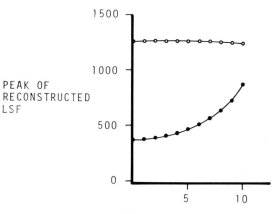

RADIAL DISTANCE FROM CR, cm

Fɪɢ. 4.13. Peak values in the reconstruction of a line source at different radial distances from the centre of rotation *CR* in air (○) and in a tissue equivalent phantom (●). The detection system was a gamma camera with 15 cm between collimator and centre of rotation.

importance, and the scheme based on the uniform distribution correction factor and an experimentally determined value of μ forms a practical system which seems to cope well with widely distributed sources such as are found in clinical practice.

4.4.3.3   Clinical application

Using such an approach, useful clinical results have been obtained in both head and body section scanning with 99m-Tc labelled compounds (Fig. 4.14). A particular benefit of transverse section imaging of the head is undoubtedly due to the unique display of the brain as symmetrical right and left halves which should be identical, thus eliminating some of the "anatomical noise" which is present when a large volume is projected and superimposed as in conventional images. Nowhere else in the body can this be achieved.

The rotating gamma camera has proved useful for transverse section imaging, using parallel-hole collimators. Images are recorded digitally, at each of a series of angles around the patient, and from these data, transverse section images can be reconstructed anywhere within the camera field of view, a considerable advantage and saving on time. Furthermore, since all the transverse planes are available, any single plane (x, y), (x, z), (y, z) or oblique can be extracted and full three-dimensional display is possible.

The practical difficulties of conventional emission imaging are compounded in tomography. Significant artefacts in the reconstruction are

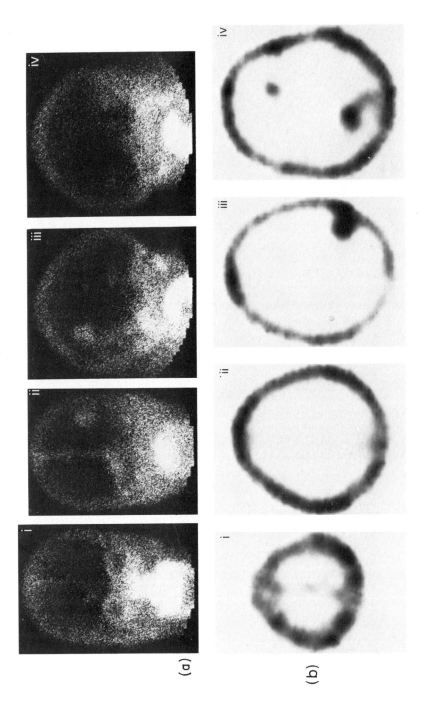

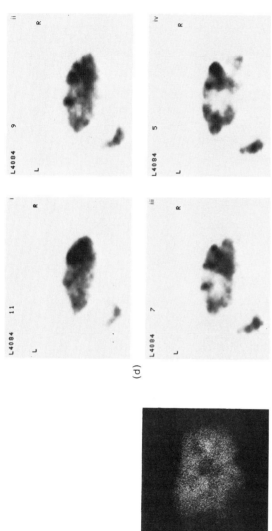

(d)

(c)

FIG. 4.14. (a) Plane views of a 99m-Tc pertechnetate brain study. (i) Anterior, (ii) posterior, (iii) right lateral and (iv) left lateral. There are two lesions on the right side, a large one in the posterior region and a smaller one lying anteriorly. (b) Four tomographic transaxial sections produced with a multi-detector scanning system (Gemmell *et al.*, 1982). Anterior is at the top of each image. Section (i) is taken through the top of the brain, while (iv) is near the base of the brain. The posterior abnormality is clearly seen on section (iii) and the anterior one on section (iv). In the posterior of section (iv) activity is seen in the transverse sinus, a normal feature. (c) Anterior plane view of a liver study showing multiple metastatic deposits. (d) Transaxial sections taken with a rotating gamma camera. Section (i) is through the upper part of the liver and section (iv) through the lower part. A large abnormality, an area showing on uptake of the radiopharmaceutical, is seen in (iii) and (iv) and smaller abnormalities in all sections. The spleen is seen posteriorly on the left side.

109

produced by inconsistency in the data arising potentially from many sources: patient movement, radionuclide movement, non-linearities and subsequent non-uniformity over the camera detector surface, mis-alignment of the measured projection and the assumed projection and poor counting statistics. The requirement of high, uniform resolution at depth is at variance with the high sensitivity collimators currently used for conventional camera imaging. The rotation of a large gamma camera in a circular orbit around the patient, with some clearance between patient and camera, necessitates quite large distances between the camera and the axis of rotation with subsequent severe loss of resolution. Elliptical orbits and body contour following are ways of improving this situation (Blum, 1983). However, preliminary studies have indicated the usefulness of the camera for transverse section imaging, and many systems are commercially available.

Multiple-detector systems, aimed at improving the relatively poor sensitivity of the early dual-detector scanner system, have also been developed (Kuhl *et al.*, 1976; Gemmell *et al.*, 1982). Increasing the number of detectors will improve the efficiency, and, provided matched detectors are available, the uniformity of sensitivity throughout the section need not suffer. One manufacturer (Union Carbide–Cleon Corporation) produced a multi-detector tomographic scanner with very large crystals and relatively short-focus collimators (Stoddart and Stoddart, 1979). The unique scanning motion utilised (Fig. 4.15) ensured that each point in the reconstruction plane emitted gamma-rays into almost a 180° arc of crystal with the same geometric efficiency, for a short period of the total data collection

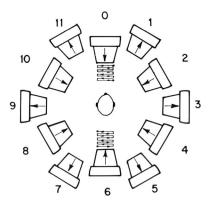

Fig. 4.15. Unique scanning motion of the multi-detector "Cleon imager". The detectors move in pairs: when one pair increments towards the centre, the adjacent pair increments away from the centre. A large crystal area is thus exposed to the section and a system with high sensitivity results.

time. An image acquired in this way is very similar to the back-projected image described earlier, and similar deconvolution techniques can be applied. This approach was unfortunately short-lived and the equipment is no longer marketed, although further research is in progress (Moore *et al.*, 1982).

A multi-detector single-photon tomography system with dynamic capability has been developed for measurements of regional cerebral blood flow (Kanno and Lassen, 1979), and other systems have been proposed. Much originality and ingenuity has been demonstrated in the design of these instruments. However, they are highly specialised and it would appear that the rotating gamma-camera-based systems are the best option for the majority of nuclear medicine departments.

4.5 Positron annihilation photon tomography

In contrast to the single-photon techniques described earlier, positron annihilation photons have some unique properties which appear advantageous in emission tomography, although much of what has been said still applies.

Following annihilation of a positron–electron pair, conservation of momentum requires that the energy appears as two very nearly oppositely directed photons, each of 511 keV. Coincident detection of these two photons in a pair of opposed detectors thus establishes the line on which the positron came to rest; conventional lead absorption collimators are not needed, leading to increased geometric efficiency and sensitivity.

With a circular array of individual scintillation crystals (Fig 4.16) coincident detection in any pair of crystals is possible. The array remains stationary and coincidence circuitry yields data corresponding to line integrals over all possible angles simultaneously. However, there are angular sampling problems and a limited degree of movement is necessary (Budinger *et al.*, 1979).

In the commercially available ECAT II (EG & G, Ltd.) there are 66 individual sodium iodide detectors, in a hexagonal arrangement around a single transverse section plane (Fig. 4.17). Each detector operates in coincidence with any one of the 11 detectors in the opposite bank. The detectors translate along the side of the hexagon to achieve a finer linear sampling, and the whole configuration also rotates stepwise to achieve finer angular sampling. A translate–rotate sequence is thus required to obtain a set of line integrals for reconstruction.

Figure 4.18 illustrates a fundamentally important difference between single-photon and annihilation photon tomography. A point source of

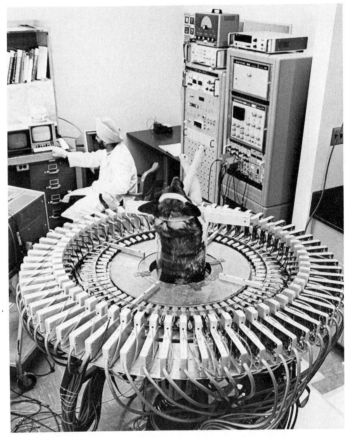

Fig. 4.16. Experimental circular array positron emission tomograph.

positron-emitting material is situated at depth x_1 relative to one detector and x_2 relative to the opposite detector. The probability of a photon reaching detector 1 is proportional to $\exp(-\mu x_1)$ and likewise the probability of a photon reaching detector 2 is proportional to $\exp(-\mu x_2)$. The probability of annihilation photons reaching both detectors and producing a coincident event is, therefore, proportional to the product $\exp(-\mu x_1)$ $\exp(-\mu x_2)$ which is independent of position between the two detectors. The coincidence count rate is, thus, dependent only on the total path length within the attenuating medium. Also, the solid angle efficiency for a pair of opposed detectors is relatively constant along the line joining the two detectors; thus, the conditions of parallel geometry referred to earlier are more appropriate than for single-photon systems. For both these reasons, the line integral of the activity along the line joining the two

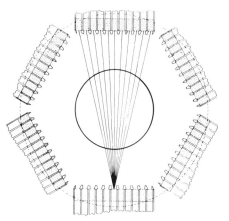

FIG. 4.17. Hexagonal array positron emission tomograph. There are 11 separate detectors on each side of the hexagon. Each detector looks to any of the opposite 11 for a coincident event.

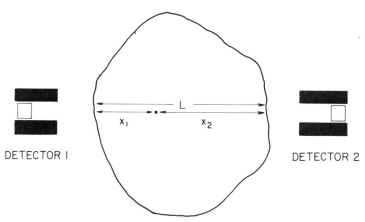

FIG. 4.18. Diagrammatic representation of coincidence detection. The coincidence counting rate from a discrete source is independent of the depth of the source and dependent only on the total path length L.

detectors can thus be more accurately inferred and in place of Eq. (4.9) we have an equation of the form

$$\frac{\text{CDR}}{f} = \int_L g(x, y)\, dy$$

where CDR is the coincidence detection rate and f the attenuation factor for 511-keV photons along the total path length L. Again several methods have been devised for estimating f. An external pre-calibrated source of positron-emitting material placed between one of the detectors and the patient can be used to measure experimentally the attenuation factor for each projection. A pre-calibrated ring source can be counted first with no patient present and then with the patient in position (before the radiopharmaceutical is administered). The ratio of the coincident event rates with/without the patient is the required factor f for each pair of crystals.

Potentially then the positron method should be more efficient and should yield quantitatively more exact reconstructions of radionuclide distributions. The biologically interesting elements carbon, nitrogen and oxygen have short-lived positron emitting radionuclides, so high activities can be administered to patients and functional studies on changing distributions are possible in tomographic mode, with suitably rapid instrumentation.

However, the technological problems are considerable. A very high background exists due to random coincidences. To reduce the random coincidence count rate, some degree of collimation is normally employed, using heavy lead shields. Additional electronic circuits are also required to monitor the random events and attempt to derive the true coincidence rate (Hoffman *et al.*, 1981). Futhermore, short-lived positron-emitting radionuclides can only be used close to a medical cyclotron and while the short physical half-life suggests that high activities may be administered, the emitted positrons have high kinetic energy which is transferred to the surrounding tissues before annihilation takes place, contributing a radiation dose similar to beta particles of equal energy (Feller *et al.*, 1979). In practice, the radiation doses from compounds of 11-C, 13-N and 15-O are likely to be of the same order of magnitude as the doses from 99m-Tc compounds, on a unit activity basis. In the immediate future, positron emission tomography is more likely to remain a sophisticated and highly specialised research methodology, rather than become a routine technique practised in the majority of nuclear medicine departments.

4.6 Concluding remarks

Single-photon emission tomography is now used widely in nuclear medicine departments, the rotating gamma camera being the most popular instrument. While this instrument may not be ideal for tomography, for example the deterioration of resolution with distance from the collimator face compares poorly with the near depth-independent characteristics which can be achieved with scanning devices, the benefit of having a device which can also be used for conventional imaging is a significant advantage over the purpose-built tomographic imager. Even a rotating gantry is not absolutely necessary since many useful tomographic studies can be carried out by a camera equipped with a rotating slant-hole or a multi-pinhole collimator.

Recent improvements in the quality of rotating camera images have been achieved by designing the camera head shielding to allow the camera to be positioned closer to the patient and by using rotation movements which follow the body contours rather than a simple circular orbit around the patient.

The potential value of tomography for providing accurate quantitative information on the radiopharmaceutical distribution is still not realised mainly due to the problem of correcting for attenuation. Improvements may result from more sophisticated reconstruction algorithms but, at present, it seems unlikely that there will be significant advances.

While the facility to perform tomography may be widely available, all too often the opinion is expressed that the technique has not been shown to have sufficient clinical value to warrant the extra time and effort needed. Several clinical trials have been reported, mostly designed to determine if more lesions can be detected with tomography, but the results are not impressive (DeLand and Shih, 1984). Small improvements have been noted for brain tomography, but they are negligible for the liver. However, trials are also required of the potential value of the tomographic image in confirming the presence of a lesion suspected from the plane view, and the value of the information tomography gives about size and location of lesions needs to be assessed critically.

Positron-annihilation photon tomography overcomes several of the limitations of single-photon tomography, conventional collimation not being necessary, and more accurate quantitation of the radiopharmaceutical is possible. Its major drawback is cost, not only of the imager but also the cyclotron. Costs may be reduced with cheap, easily run 'minicyclotrons' and, perhaps, low-cost imagers such as the multi-wire proportional counter devices (see Section 6.2.2).

References

Anger, H. O. (1969). Multi-plane tomographic gamma ray scanner. *In* "Medical Radioisotope Scintigraphy", Vol. 1, pp. 203–216. IAEA, Vienna.

Blum, A. S. (1983). Improving SPECT image quality by body contour-following. *In* "Emission Computed Tomography" (P. D. Esser, ed.), pp. 163–173. Society of Nuclear Medicine, New York.

Bracewell, R. N. and Riddle, A. C. (1967). Inversion of fan-beam scans in radio-astronomy. *Astrophys. J.* **150**, 427–434.

Budinger, T. F., Derenzo, S. E., Gullberg, G. T. and Huesman, R. H. (1979). Trends and prospects for circular ring positron cameras. *IEEE Trans. Nucl. Sci.* **NS-26**, 2742–2745.

Chesler, D. A. and Riederer, S. J. (1975). Ripple suppression during reconstruction in transverse tomography. *Phys. Med. Biol.* **20**, 632–636.

Cormack, A. M. (1973). Reconstruction of densities from their projections, with applications in radiological physics. *Phys. Med. Biol.* **18**, 195–207.

DeLand, F. H. and Shih, W. J. (1984). The status of SPECT in tumor diagnosis. *J. Nucl. Med.* **25**, 1375–1379.

Feller, P. A., Sodd, V. J. and Nishiyama, H. (1979). Absorbed dose comparisons: positron emitters 11-C, 13-N and 15-O versus gamma ray emitters. *Med. Phys.* **6**, 221–223.

Gemmell, H. G., Dendy, P. P., Pitt, W. R., Evans, N. T. S. and Mallard, J. R. (1982). Physical criteria for the performance of tomographic imaging systems. *In* "Nuclear Medicine and Biology" (C. Raynaud, ed.). Vol. 1, pp. 476–479. Pergamon Press, Paris.

Gullberg, G. T. (1979). The attenuated Radon transform. Ph.D. Thesis, University of California, Berkeley. LBL-7486.

Hoffman, E. J., Huang, S. C., Phelps, M. E. and Kuhl, E. E. (1981). Quantitation in positron computed emission tomography 4: effect of accidental coincidence. *J. Comp. Assist. Tomogr.* **5**, 391–400.

Kanno, I. and Lassen, N. A. (1979). Two methods for calculating regional cerebral blood flow from emission computed tomography of inert gas concentrations. *J. Comp. Assist. Tomogr.* **3**, 71–76.

Keyes, W. I. (1976). A practical approach to transverse section gamma ray imaging. *Br. J. Radiol.* **49**, 62–70.

Keyes, W. I. (1979). Current status of single photon emission computerised tomography. *IEEE Trans. Nucl. Sci.* **NS-26**, 2751–2755.

Kuhl, D. E. (1964). A clinical radioisotope scanner for cylindrical and section scanning. *In* Medical Radioisotope Scanning", Vol. 1, pp. 273–289. IAEA, Vienna.

Kuhl, D. E. and Edwards, R. Q. (1963). Image separation radioisotope scanning. *Radiology* **80**, 653–661.

Kuhl, D. E., Edwards, R. Q. and Ricci, A. R. (1976). The Mark IV system for radionuclide computed tomography of the brain. *Radiology* **121**, 405–413.

Meuhllehner, G. (1971). A tomographic scintillation camera. *Phys. Med. Biol.* **16**, 87–96.

Moore, S. C., Parker, J. A., Zimmerman, R. E., Budinger, T. F. and Holman, B. L. (1982). The effect of angular sampling on image quality of the Harvard multi-detector ECT brain scanner. *In* "Nuclear Medicine and Biology" (C. Raynaud, ed.), Vol. 1, pp. 531–534. Pergamon Press, Paris.

Rowe, R. W. (1979). Quantitative single photon emission computerised transaxial tomography. Ph.D. Thesis, University of Aberdeen.

Rowe, R. W. and Keyes, W. I. (1979). Comparison of scanner and camera systems for quantitative single photon emission tomography. *IEEE Trans. Nucl. Sci.* **NS-26**, 2768–2771.

Smith, P. R., Peters, T. M. and Bates, R. H. T. (1973). Image reconstruction from finite numbers of projections. *J. Phys. A* **6**, 361–382.

Stoddart, H. F. and Stoddart, H. A. (1979). A new development in single gamma transaxial tomography. *IEEE Trans. Nucl. Sci.* **NS-26**, 2710–2712.

Vainstein, B. K. (1970). Finding the structure of objects from projections. *Kristallografiya* **15**, 894–902 [*Sov. Phys.—Crystallogr. (Engl. Transl.)* **15**, 781–787 (1971)].

Vogel, R. A., Kirsch, D., LeFree, M. and Steele, P. (1978). A new method of multiplanar emission tomography using a seven pinhole collimator and an Anger scintillation camera. *J. Nucl. Med.* **19**, 648–654.

Zenari, A., Scrimger, J. W. and Hooper, R. (1983). An assessment of the physical properties of a multiplane tomographic imager. *Phys. Med. Biol.* **28**, 1235–1249.

Chapter 5

Measurement of Imaging Device Performance

5.1 Introduction

The specification of the performance of an imaging device, whilst of paramount importance, has in practice proved difficult to achieve. There are two main situations in which such measurements are necessary: in comparing the performance of imaging devices, and in maintaining a check on the performance of one particular instrument.

The former problem is, for most practising medical physicists, one of comparing the merits of different versions of one type of instrument, usually a gamma camera, produced by different manufacturers. This has been somewhat simplified by the introduction of standards for performance specification by the National Electrical Manufacturer's Association (NEMA) in the United States and the International Electrotechnical Commission (IEC) in Europe, details of which can be found in papers by Muehllehner *et al.* (1981) and Sano (1980). The problem of comparing the performance of different types of device has long proved a challenge and will not be considered here in any detail.

The second situation in which performance needs to be measured is in quality control. Not surprisingly, the difference between the two problems is mainly one of emphasis rather than choice of parameters measured.

Both the NEMA and IEC standards are unsuitable for use in the hospital environment and tests for both performance assessment and quality control have been proposed by the Hospital Physicists' Association (HPA) (Horton *et al.*, 1978) in the United Kingdom and a Bureau of Radiological

Health Group (Paras, 1976, 1980, Hine *et al.*, 1977, 1979) in the United States.

Perhaps the two most important parameters to consider are spatial resolution and sensitivity, while the need to maintain linearity requires both spatial and temporal linearity to be examined. Nonstationarity, i.e. variations in performance across the detector face, are best demonstrated by the non-uniformity of a flood image. Finally energy resolution is also important since the relatively low-energy gamma photons used in clinical imaging make discrimination against small-angle Compton scatter difficult. In the following sections these factors will be considered in detail, typical values for the different parameters being given in Table 5.1.

Most work on performance is concerned with gamma cameras and, to a lesser extent, rectilinear scanners, but recently it has become obvious that parameters need to be modified when applied to tomographic systems and these will be considered separately in Section 5.8.

TABLE 5.1. Typical performance parameters.[a]

Intrinsic spatial resolution—NEMA		
3.6 mm FWHM,	6.76 mm FWTM	(UFOV)
3.5 mm FWHM,	6.58 mm FWTM	(CFOV)

Intrinsic FWHM and FWTM—IEC		
3.5 mm FWHM,	6.68 mm FWTM	(x axis)
3.6 mm FWHM,	6.72 mm FWTM	(y axis)
3.6 mm FWHM,	6.75 mm FWTM	(45° edge)

System spatial resolution—NEMA (ultrafine collimator)			
9.1 mm FWHM,	18.61 mm FWTM	(CFOV)	air
9.8 mm FWHM,	24.15 mm FWTM	(CFOV)	lucite

Intrinsic energy resolution—NEMA	
12.4%	FWHM at 140 keV

Energy resolution (collimator plus scatter)—IEC	
14.3%	FWHM

Intrinsic flood field uniformity—NEMA		
±6.7%	Integral uniformity	(UFOV)
±3.4%	Integral uniformity	(CFOV)
±1.6%	Differential uniformity	(UFOV)
±0.8%	Differential uniformity	(CFOV)
±3.8%	Point source sensitivity variation	

TABLE 5.1 (*cont.*)

	System non-uniformity—IEC
0%	Pixels within ±15%
0%	Pixels within ±10%
15.8%	Pixels within ±5%
6.7%	Maximum deviation
2.3%	Maximum differential uniformity

	Intrinsic count-rate performance—NEMA	
40,725 cps	at the 20% loss point	
85,575 cps	maximum count rate	
3.9 mm	FWHM resolution at 75,000 cps	(UFOV)
3.8 mm	FWHM resolution at 75,000 cps	(CFOV)
7.3 mm	FWTM resolution at 75,000 cps	(UFOV)
7.0 mm	FWTM resolution at 75,000 cps	(CFOV)
±7.3%	Integral uniformity at 75,000 cps	(UFOV)
±3.8%	Integral uniformity at 75,000 cps	(CFOV)
±1.8%	Differential uniformity at 75,000 cps	(UFOV)
±0.9%	Differential uniformity at 75,000 cps	(CFOV)

	System sensitivity—NEMA
350 counts/(min μCi)	(General purpose collimator and 99m-Tc)

	Plane sensitivity—IEC
1.59×10^{-4} counts/(sec Bq)	(General purpose collimator and 99m-Tc)

	Intrinsic spatial linearity—NEMA	
8.4 mm	Absolute linearity displacement	(UFOV)
3.8 mm	Absolute linearity displacement	(CFOV)
5.3 mm	Standard deviation	(UFOV)
1.4 mm	Standard deviation	(CFOV)

[a] UFOV is the useful field of view, the full field of view of the collimator. CFOV is the central field of view, 75% of the diameter of the UFOV. Adapted from Sano (1980).

5.2   Sensitivity

Sensitivity is a measure of the proportion of emitted gamma rays which are used to form the image. Geometric efficiency, used earlier in the discussion about collimators, is only one of the factors affecting device sensitivity. The sensitivity of the detector itself and the proportion of gamma rays accepted by the pulse height analyser must also be taken into account.

Sensitivity can be measured by flooding all the collimator holes with gamma rays using a plane source of activity larger than the collimator's field of view, and then measuring the resulting count rate. Plane source sensitivity or absolute sensitivity S_A is defined as

$$S_A = \frac{\text{recorded count rate}}{\text{area of the field of view of collimator}} \Big/ \frac{\text{source activity}}{\text{source surface area}}$$

(5.1)

and has units of cps Bq^{-1}.

The main advantage of this measure is that provided the source size is larger than the field of view, absolute sensitivity will be independent of source–collimator distance in air. Care must be taken that the source is thin enough to avoid self-attenuation and the count rate must be sufficiently low to minimise data losses (see Section 5.4). In practice a source thickness of 5 mm and a count rate not exceeding 15 kcps are usually satisfactory.

Absolute sensitivity represents an average value of the sensitivity over the field of view and so is of greatest relevance when sensitivity is spatially invariant, as is the case for a gamma camera fitted with a parallel-hole collimator. In these circumstances any shape of source may be used provided that it is contained within the collimator's field of view and subject to the preceding restrictions on thickness and count rate. Sensitivity measured in this way is known as relative sensitivity S_R and can be defined as

$$S_R = \frac{\text{recorded count rate}}{\text{activity in source}}$$

(5.2)

NEMA uses a 10-cm-diameter plane source positioned at the centre of the field of view, while the HPA recommends a square source of side length 10 cm. If a point or line source is employed, then sensitivity can be measured at the same time as spatial resolution (see next section). Sources other than the large flood plane source measure relative sensitivity over only part of the detector area, and in the presence of non-uniformities (Section 5.6) this may bias the results.

As already mentioned, sensitivity depends upon the pulse height spectrum, and this will vary with the amount of scatter present. In the IEC recommendations, relative sensitivity measurements are made with a 10-cm-diameter cylinder surrounded by several centimetres of Perspex to give scattered radiation.

Relative sensitivity is useful where sensitivity changes across the field of view, as when converging, diverging or pinhole collimators are used, since it allows sensitivity to be expressed as a function of spatial position. The point source is particularly useful for this measurement.

Moving detector devices pose a slightly different problem. As the point spread function (PSF) of the focussed collimator of the rectilinear scanner is produced by measuring the variation in count rate as the scanner moves across the point source, it will also show how relative sensitivity varies. Sets of unnormalised PSFs, as in Fig. 3.3, can thus demonstrate variations of both sensitivity and spatial resolution. The area under the PSF [or line spread function (LSF)] gives the absolute sensitivity, and when attenuation is negligible it is invariant of distance of source from collimator face (see also Section 2.1.4).

Comparing a moving detector device with a stationary one also poses problems. Causer and Mallard (1974) proposed that sensitivity could be measured for the rectilinear scanner by recording the count rate from a plane source larger than the collimator's field of view and calculating

$$\text{Unit plane sensitivity} = \frac{\text{count rate}}{\text{area of scan}} \Big/ \frac{\text{source activity}}{\text{source area}} \qquad (5.3)$$

This requires that the intended scan area be specified, but if this can be done in a meaningful way then a measure of sensitivity comparable with absolute sensitivity is obtained.

5.3 Spatial resolution

Spatial resolution can be measured objectively by examining the response of the device to an impulse input signal produced by either a point or line source of radioactivity (Section 2.1.4). The full width at half-maximum height (FWHM) of the PSF or LSF (Fig. 5.1) is frequently used as a measure of resolution, the resolution index, since it is claimed (MacIntyre et al., 1969) that two line sources separated by this distance can just be resolved. In optics this is known as the Rayleigh criterion.

Spatial resolution may refer either to total system resolution, i.e., detector plus collimator, or intrinsic resolution when the effect of the collimator is not considered. In the first case line sources can be easily constructed from nylon cannulas of internal diameter less than, say, 2 mm. When intrinsic measurements are made it is necessary to produce an image of the line in the detector crystal without the aid of the collimator. This can be done either by placing a lead plate with a narrow slit on the detector face and imaging it by transmission (the approach adopted by NEMA) or by placing a line source in a slit in a lead block, the slit collimating the source.

A single value such as the FWHM is obviously an incomplete specification of the LSF, and in both the NEMA and IEC standards the full width at tenth-maximum height (FWTM) is also quoted. This is particularly

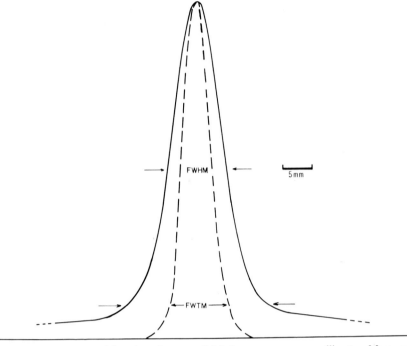

FIG. 5.1. Line spread functions for a parallel hole gamma camera collimator. Measurements are made with the line source on top of the camera face (dashed curve) and 10 cm deep in tissue equivalent material (solid curve). The full width at half-maximum height (FWHM) and full width at tenth-maximum height (FWTM) are shown by the arrows.

pertinent since scattered radiation mainly affects the tails of the LSF, as can be seen in Fig. 5.1.

While the LSF provides a complete description of resolution, it is not in a very convenient form. If it can be assumed that the system is linear, then the system transfer function (STF) can be derived from the Fourier transform of the PSF or LSF

$$\text{STF}(f_x, f_y) = \int\int \text{PSF}(x, y)[\cos 2\pi(f_x x + f_y y) \tag{5.4}$$

$$+ i \ \sin 2\pi(f_x x + f_y y)]\, dx\, dy \bigg/ \int\int \text{PSF}(x, y)\, dx\, dy$$

$$\text{STF}(f_x) = \int \text{LSF}(x)\,(\cos 2\pi f_x x + i \sin 2\pi f_x x)\, dx \bigg/ \int \text{LSF}(x)\, dx \tag{5.5}$$

The STF can be considered as consisting of two parts:

(i) the modulation transfer function (MTF) = $|STF|$, i.e.,

$$MTF(f_x) = \left[\left(\int LSF(x) \cos 2\pi f_x x \, dx \right)^2 + \left(\int LSF(x) \sin 2\pi f_x x \, dx \right)^2 \right]^{1/2} \Bigg/ \int LSF(x) \, dx \qquad (5.6)$$

(ii) the phase transfer function (PTF) where

$$PTF(f_x) = \tan^{-1} \left\{ \int LSF(x) \sin 2\pi f_x x \, dx \Bigg/ \int LSF(x) \cos 2\pi f_x x \, dx \right\} \qquad (5.7)$$

In many practical cases the LSF is symmetrical about its peak and, assuming that the origin of the coordinate system is centred on the peak, then the imaginary part of the STF (i.e, the sine term) becomes zero. This simplifies system description, since the PTF is then 0 or π and the MTF can be calculated from the LSF by the equation

$$MTF(f_x) = \int LSF(x) \cos(2\pi f_x x) \, dx \Bigg/ \int LSF(x) \, dx \qquad (5.8)$$

The MTFs corresponding to the LSFs of Fig. 5.1 are given in Fig. 5.2. By definition the MTF will be positive and range between unity and zero, its value representing the fidelity with which that particular spatial frequency is reproduced by the device (Fig. 5.3). An ideal imaging system would have an MTF of unity at all frequencies. In Fig. 5.2 the degradation of resolution with increasing depth in scattering material is shown by the drop in the value of the MTF at a given frequency. The IEC recommends that MTF be quoted for each collimator, but MTF is not used by NEMA.

Resolution can also be assessed subjectively by visual inspection of a test-pattern image. Two of the most common patterns, the quadrant bar phantom and Anger phantom (Anger, 1973), are shown in Fig. 5.4. The bar phantom consists of lead bars 9.6, 6.4, 4.8 and 4 mm in width and 2 mm thick imaged by placing a flood source behind it. Resolution is judged from the minimum resolvable bar spacing (see also Section 5.9.1). The Anger phantom is made from holes of 5, 4, 3.5, 3, 2.5 and 2 mm in diameter in a lead sheet and is also imaged by placing a flood source behind it. As relatively few photons are transmitted, it is only suitable for measuring intrinsic resolution.

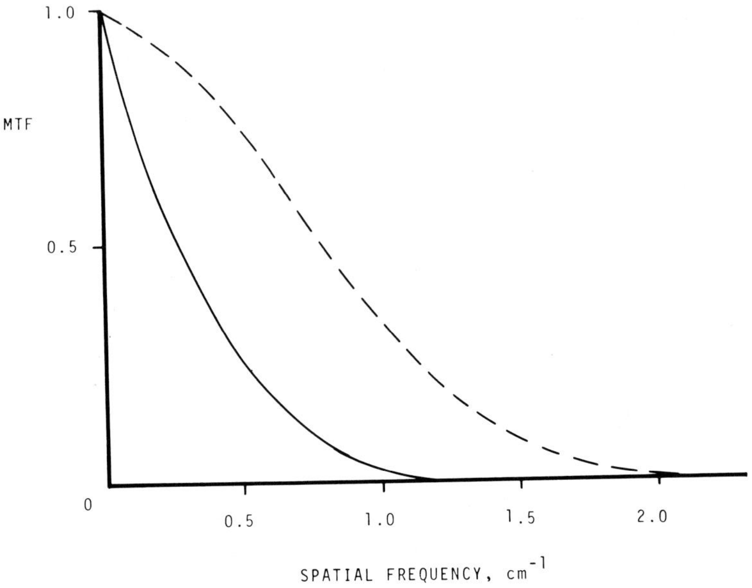
1.0
MTF
0.5
0
0.5
1.0
1.5
2.0
SPATIAL FREQUENCY, cm^{-1}

FIG. 5.2. Modulation transfer functions corresponding to the line spread functions of Fig. 5.1.

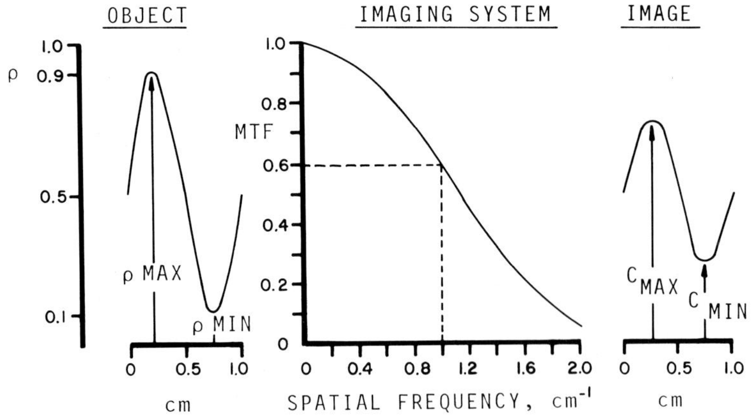
OBJECT
IMAGING SYSTEM
IMAGE
ρ
1.0
0.9
0.5
0.1
ρ MAX
ρ MIN
0
0.5
1.0
cm
MTF
1.0
0.8
0.6
0.4
0.2
0
0
0.4
0.8
1.2
1.6
2.0
SPATIAL FREQUENCY, cm^{-1}
C MAX
C MIN
0
0.5
1.0
cm

FIG. 5.3. Variation of activity ρ in the object shown as a sine wave with a frequency of 1 cycle/cm and a modulation $(\rho_{MAX} - \rho_{MIN})/(\rho_{MAX} + \rho_{MIN})$ of 0.8. The MTF of the imaging system at this frequency is 0.6, resulting in a modulation of the imaged sine wave of $0.6 \times 0.8 = 0.48$. A complex object can be considered as the weighted sum of sine waves of various frequencies, each of which will be modified by the imaging system according to its MTF. [Figure reproduced by kind permission of Professor J. R. Mallard.]

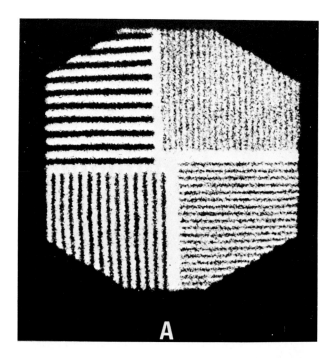

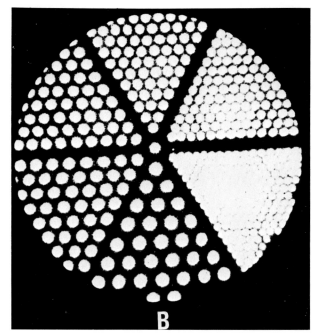

Fig. 5.4. Test patterns for spatial resolution. (a) The image of a quadrant bar phantom. The widths of the bars are 4, 4.8, 6.4 and 9.6 mm. (b) The image of the Anger phantom. The hole diameters are 2, 2.5, 3, 3.5, 4 and 5 mm.

5.4 Temporal resolution

For accurate imaging of the distribution of radioactivity in a patient, it is important to ensure that device performance is unaffected by the count rate. In practice, at high count rates both the count rate recorded by the device and spatial information in the image become distorted.

The relationship between input and output count rate is governed by the temporal resolution, sometimes referred to as the dead time, of the device. Imaging systems can be categorised as paralyzable, non-paralyzable or a mixture of the two (Evans, 1955). In a paralyzable system an interval of at least D sec must elapse between successive counts; an event occurring within this interval causes this dead-time to be extended by a further D sec. In contrast, while the non-paralyzable system also will not record events arriving within D sec of each other, this interval is not extended should an event occur within it.

For the paralyzable system, the observed (i.e., recorded) count rate and the true count rate T are related by

$$O = Te^{-TD} \tag{5.9}$$

which at low count rates $(TD \ll 1)$ becomes

$$O = T(1 - TD) \tag{5.10}$$

With increasing values of T, the observed count rate gradually reaches a maximum value

$$O_{max} = 1/eD \tag{5.11}$$

after which it actually decreases.

In the non-paralyzable system,

$$O = T(1 - OD) \tag{5.12}$$

which at low count rates behaves as the paralyzable system [Eq. (5.10)] but at high count rates approaches a maximum value O_{max} asymptotically, where

$$O_{max} = 1/D \tag{5.13}$$

At its maximum the system is simply recording a count once every D sec.

Many gamma cameras, particularly when connected to data processing equipment, behave as a mixture of paralyzable and non-paralyzable systems (Muehllehner and Colsher, 1983).

In practice, temporal resolution is complicated by a dependence upon the energy spectrum of input gamma photons, the window width of the pulse height analyser and the spatial distribution of the gamma rays. The simplest method of measurement is to place a point source of radioactivity about 1 m away from the uncollimated detector so as to flood the detector uniformly. The recorded count rate is then plotted as a function of the activity of the source. At low activities the curve is linear and so a calibration factor giving the expected count rate as a function of source activity can be calculated. Using this factor, the recorded count rate can be plotted against expected input count rate (Fig. 3.19).

If it is assumed that the camera behaves as a paralyzable system, at least over the range of clinically relevant count rates, then the dead-time value D used with Eq. (5.9) completely specifies temporal resolution. A more useful approach though, and one which is adopted in practice, is to specify performance in terms of the count rate corresponding to a given percentage count loss. NEMA recommends the input count rate which produces a 20% count loss. The HPA and IEC, in contrast, propose that recorded, rather than input, count rates be used. The HPA suggests using the value which is 90% of the expected count rate, while IEC uses the 80% value. In addition, HPA and NEMA also give the maximum recorded count rate O_{max}.

Varying the activity in a point source can be a lengthy task, liable to introduce errors. The simplest alternative is to let the activity decay, but this requires measurements to be made over many hours for a radionuclide like 99m-Tc. In the NEMA measurements calibrated sheets of copper are used to absorb the gamma rays, although this may also alter the energy spectrum.

The maximum recorded count rate alone can be found simply by moving the point source towards the camera, this being the procedure adopted by NEMA.

If it can be assumed that the device is paralyzable, then the two-vial method (Adams *et al.*, 1974) can be used to measure dead time. Two vials containing approximately equal amounts of activity are used such that when imaged together the input count rate is high enough to cause about 20% loss of counts. If R_A is the count rate produced by vial A, R_B by vial B, and R_{A+B} when imaged together, then

$$D = \left(\frac{2R_{A+B}}{(R_A + R_B)^2}\right) \ln\left(\frac{R_A + R_B}{R_{A+B}}\right) \tag{5.14}$$

The method is simple to perform and is used in the NEMA recommendations to ascertain the input count rate producing a 20% count loss.

The energy spectrum of the gamma photons can be more closely approximated to that encountered clinically by introducing scatter material. Figure 5.5 shows the phantom recommended by the HPA group for this purpose, measurements being made with a collimator on the camera. Both the energy spectrum and photon spatial distribution are different

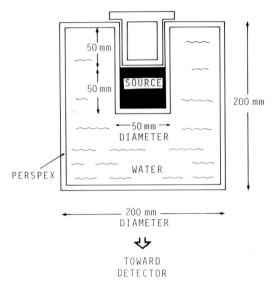

Fig. 5.5. HPA phantom for measuring temporal resolution.

from the flood method and the effect on temporal resolution can be seen in Fig. 5.6. For example, the input count rate causing a 10% data loss is 45 kcps when the flood method is used but only 17 kcps with the HPA phantom. A similar phantom is used in the IEC standards. Adams *et al.* (1978) have also adapted the two-vial method to include scattering material.

The effect of temporal resolution on the quality of images has been demonstrated in several papers (Murphy *et al.*, 1977; Strand and Larsson,

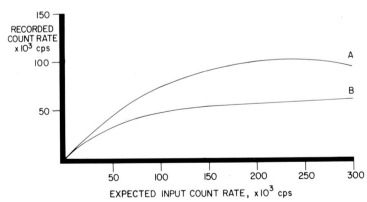

Fig. 5.6. Temporal resolution curves measured either by using a point source of radioactivity to flood the uncollimated detector (curve A) or by imaging the HPA phantom shown in Fig. 5.5 (curve B).

1978; Guldberg and Rossing, 1978). NEMA recommends that intrinsic spatial resolution and flood uniformity should be measured at a count rate of 75 kcps, i.e., close to the maximum recordable rate. IEC suggests measuring orthogonal profiles through the image of the source used for temporal resolution measurements at count rates of 50, 25 and 1 kcps.

5.5 Spatial linearity

While spatial resolution defines the sharpness of an image, linearity measures positional distortion. Such distortions must be comparable with system resolution to affect a clinical image, but unfortunately much smaller non-linearities will cause non-uniformities in regions of otherwise uniform count density (Muehllehner et al., 1980). The problem of non-uniformity is discussed in the next section. To assess such small deviations requires careful measurements which must be made without a collimator if the necessary resolution is to be achieved.

Linearity can be appreciated by a visual examination of a test-pattern image, a regular array of lines or holes such as in Fig. 5.7. Quantitative

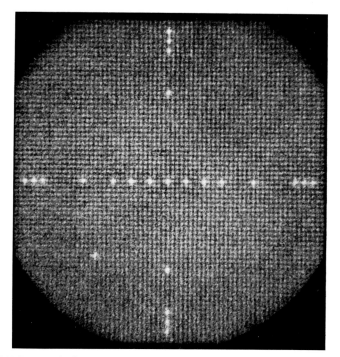

FIG. 5.7. Image of a linearity phantom consisting of an array of parallel lines of equally spaced holes.

measurements require not only the actual position of lines or holes to be determined but also calculation of their true (undistorted) position.

In the NEMA measurements a lead plate with 1-mm-wide parallel slits at 3 cm separation is used. An image is taken with the slits parallel to the X axis and then to the Y axis of the detector. The position of the peak of each slit profile is found by interpolation and the correct position of the lines is determined from a least-squares fit using the peak positions. Absolute linearity is defined as the maximum displacement from the expected position and differential linearity as the standard deviation of the peak positions about the expected positions.

The HPA recommends using four collimated line sources arranged in a rectangle with sides parallel to the X and Y axes. Linearity is quoted in terms of maximum and minimum deviations expressed as a percentage of line length.

5.6 Uniformity

Uniformity is a measure of the accuracy with which the device produces an image of a spatially uniform gamma-ray flux. Figure 3.17 shows an example of such an image; systematic variations in count density are apparent and, as discussed in Section 3.3.5, they are the result of changes in energy response and spatial linearity across the gamma camera's face.

It is important to measure such non-uniformities since these areas of above- or below-average count density may be confused with abnormal pathology in clinical images (Van Tuinen *et al.*, 1978). Uniformity can be assessed either directly, by analyzing the count density pattern in a flood image, or indirectly, by monitoring a parameter known to cause non-uniformity.

5.6.1 Direct methods

This is the most commonly used approach. Flood images can be produced by using a plane source of radioactivity placed on the collimated detector. A Perspex tank filled with an aqueous solution of a radionuclide or radionuclide dispersed in a plastic sheet is commonly used for this purpose. Alternatively a point source of radioactivity positioned a metre or so away from the uncollimated detector can be used. The latter method has the advantage of being simple to perform and requiring only about 5 MBq of activity. However great care must be taken to position the point source on the central axis of the detector and sufficiently far away from the detector face to give a uniform flux. For a detector with a 38-cm-diameter field of view, a point source 1.5 m away will give a flood image in which there is a 1.6% difference in photon flux between the centre and edge of the image due to the inverse square law.

The simplest and perhaps the most accurate way to judge uniformity is by visual inspection of the image. As part of a quality control procedure, however, there are advantages in supplementing this by a quantitative measure.

Quantification requires that the flood image be first digitised, and this may introduce distortions. The counts in a pixel must be high enough to minimise statistical flunctuations, and typically 10^4 counts/pixel are acquired (1% fractional standard deviation), but if a small pixel size is to be used to minimise spatial distortion this may result in an unacceptably long collection time. NEMA recommends using a point source to produce the flood image, data being acquired on a 64×64 pixel matrix with a minimum of 4000 counts/pixel. They also smooth the data (Section 8.3.1) before analyzing it.

IEC use a flood source with 2-cm-thick Perspex front and rear surfaces so that the energy spectrum of the photons producing the flood image contains a degree of scatter similar to that encountered in clinical practice.

They suggest a pixel size equal to twice the value of the FWHM of the collimator 2 cm from the face (approximately equivalent to using a 32×32 matrix) and 10^4 counts/pixel.

Sharp and Marshall (1981), in an experiment to examine the correlation between the visual impression of non-uniformity and quantitative measures of uniformity, concluded that a pixel of side 18 mm, equivalent to a 21×21 matrix, was best.

Quantitative measures of uniformity fall into three classes:

(i) Integral uniformity. This is a measure of the range of counts per pixel in the image. The HPA group suggests that it should be quoted as

$$U(+) = [(C_{MAX} - C_{AV})/C_{AV}] \times 100\% \qquad (5.15)$$

and

$$U(-) = [(C_{MIN} - C_{AV})/C_{AV}] \times 100\% \qquad (5.16)$$

where C_{MAX}, C_{MIN} and C_{AV} are the maximum, minimum and mean number of counts per pixel. IEC advises that only the larger of $U(+)$ and $U(-)$ values be quoted. NEMA defines integral uniformity as

$$[(C_{MAX} - C_{MIN})/(C_{MAX} + C_{MIN})] \times 100\% \qquad (5.17)$$

(ii) Differential uniformity. This is a measure of the maximum "contrast" in the flood image.

The HPA recommends the equation

$$(\Delta C_{MAX}/C_{AV}\Delta x) \times 100\% \qquad (5.18)$$

where ΔC_{MAX} is the maximum difference between counts in adjacent pixels and Δx is the length of a pixel side. The IEC recommended measure of differential uniformity is

$$(\Delta C_{MAX}/C_{HIGH}) \times 100\% \qquad (5.19)$$

where $C_{HIGH} - C_{LOW} = \Delta C_{MAX}$.

NEMA considers horizontal and vertical rows of five adjacent pixels, this being approximately the size of a photomultiplier tube, and defines differential uniformity as

$$[(C_{MAX} - C_{MIN})/(C_{MAX} + C_{MIN})] \times 100\% \qquad (5.20)$$

where $C_{MAX} - C_{MIN}$ represents the greatest difference between any two pixels from a row or column of five.

(iii)   Global measures. Both integral and differential uniformity measure the greatest deviations in the image but give no indication of the uniformity of the rest of the image. Several global measures have been suggested.

(a)   Coefficient of variation of counts per pixel. This is given by

$$\left[\sum_i C(i)^2 n(i) \bigg/ \sum_i n(i)\right]^{1/2} \times \frac{100}{C_{AV}} \qquad (5.21)$$

where $n(i)$ is the number of pixels with $C(i)$ counts.

(b)   Spread of differential uniformity. Sharp and Marshall (1981) suggested that, rather than use the range of contrast values to express differential uniformity, the spread of the frequency distribution of these values should be calculated as

$$\left[\sum_i \Delta C(i)^2 n(i) \bigg/ \sum_i n(i)\right]^{1/2} \times \frac{100}{\Delta x} \qquad (5.22)$$

where $n(i)$ is the number of times a difference in count density of $\Delta C(i)$ was measured between adjacent pixels.

(c)   Frequency distribution of counts per pixel. IEC proposes that the percentage of the total number of pixels whose counts exceed ± 5, ± 10 and $\pm 15\%$ of the mean value should be given.

(d)   Uniformity index. Cox and Diffey (1976) compensate for the possible effect of statistical noise on the measurement of uniformity by subtracting from the measured variance in the number of counts per pixel the variance expected from statistical (Poisson) noise, i.e., C_{AV}

$$\text{Uniformity index} = \left\{ \left[\sum_i C(i)^2 n(i) \Big/ \sum_i n(i) \right] - C_{AV} \right\}^{1/2} \times \frac{100}{C_{AV}} \quad (5.23)$$

(e) Index of uniformity. Nusynowitz and Benedetto (1979) analyse the non-uniformity of a flood image by computing the best fit plane to the image

$$Z = a + bx + cy \quad (5.24)$$

where x and y are orthogonal coordinates and a, b and c are constants. Non-uniformity is indicated if either b or c is significantly different from zero. In addition, Nusynowitz and Benedetto measure the deviations of the counts in each pixel about this plane

$$D = \left[\sum_{i=1}^{N} d(i)^2 / (N - 3) \right]^{1/2} \quad (5.25)$$

where $d(i)$ is the difference between the recorded number of counts in the ith pixel and that expected from Eq. (5.24) and N is the total number of pixels. Nusynowitz and Benedetto define an index of uniformity IOU as

$$\text{IOU} = 1 - 2D/S$$

where the plane sensitivity S is proportional to the constant a in Eq. (5.24). If IOU is less than 0.9, then uniformity is judged to be unacceptable.

5.6.2 Indirect methods

NEMA proposes that the variations in the count rate recorded when a collimated point source is moved over the detector face should be recorded. The point source sensitivity variation is given by

$$\pm [(MAX - MIN)/(MAX + MIN)] \quad (5.26)$$

where MAX and MIN are the maximum and minimum recorded count rates.

5.7 Energy resolution

Statistical variations in the measurement of the energy of a detected gamma ray (Section 2.1.3) result in the photo-peak appearing on the pulse height analyser as a bell-shaped curve rather than a single line. The width of this curve, usually taken as the FWHM, gives the energy resolution of the device. It is measured in the conventional manner using either a single-channel or a multi-channel analyser (Ross and Harris, 1969) and the FWHM is expressed as a percentage of the photo-peak energy. Since energy resolution depends upon the photo-peak energy, this value must always be quoted.

5.8 Performance measurements for tomographic systems

In a tomographic study, each point in the object is measured several times, and the final image is reconstructed from this multiplicity of measurements. There are thus additional degrees of freedom on how resolution and sensitivity may be defined and measured.

Resolution needs to be specified both within and perpendicular to the plane of the section. As a measure of resolution within the section, a line source positioned perpendicular to the plane of the section may be imaged at various radial distances from the centre of rotation (CR) of the system, either in air or within a cylindrical water phantom (see Fig. 4.12). A profile through the reconstructed image could then be used to give FWHM measurements. The reconstructed image of the source will, of course, depend on the particular algorithm used, the angular increment between views and also on the rigidity/alignment of the rotational mechanism. The image will not necessarily be circularly symmetric, due mainly to variations in the depth response of the detection system. Thus, a profile through the centre of the reconstructed image will not be unique. Ideally the variation should be small for all positions of the line source within, say, a 10-cm radius of the CR for systems designed for the head and within a 15-cm radius for whole body systems.

Typical values for the FWHM of such profiles for current systems are 10–20 mm, and the variation is usually better than ±2 mm for a properly collimated, well-adjusted system.

The resolution perpendicular to the section gives an estimate of the effective section thickness, and this can be measured using a point source. Reconstructions of the point source can be obtained at each of a number of different distances away from the plane of the section, the peak value of the reconstruction plotted against distance yielding an appropriate profile. However, since there is a variation in the depth response of the detector over the plane of the section, the radial distance of the point source from the CR influences the profile shape. A planar disc source lying parallel to the plane of the section would be more appropriate, but since such a source would be difficult to fabricate in unit density material, it has been suggested that the edge of a cylindrical source, i.e., the boundary between active and non-active cylinders, be used to obtain an "edge profile", which can then be differentiated to find the appropriate disc response profile (Flower *et al.*, 1981).

The sensitivities of the different systems in tomographic mode are, for intercomparison purposes, best measured using the total counts collected from a specific source, e.g., a cylinder uniformly filled with radioactive solution. This avoids difficulties in using the values taken from reconstructed images where arbitrary normalisations in the different reconstruction algorithms may affect the results. Since both scanning and gamma-camera systems are used for tomography, the imaged section area also needs to be specified. Single-section sensitivity (SSS) can be defined as

$$\text{SSS} \equiv \frac{\text{total counts collected in a single section}}{\text{total imaging time} \times \text{radioactivity concentration}} \tag{5.27}$$

and for a 19-cm-diameter cylinder and 34-cm-diameter section area, values of SSS between 18 and 260 counts/(sec kBq cm^3) have been measured for several systems (Flower *et al.*, 1981) with a multi-detector device producing the highest figure.

The SSS does not take into account any capability of the device to produce multiple sections simultaneously. Thus, multiple-section sensitivity (MSS) is defined as

$$\text{MSS} \equiv \frac{\text{total counts collected from all sections}}{\text{total imaging time} \times \text{radioactivity concentration}} \tag{5.28}$$

again for a specific source and imaged area. The gamma camera can produce multiple sections simultaneously, whereas single-section systems must repeat the scan for each section. Therefore, when more and more sections are considered necessary, the gamma camera eventually has the highest MSS. For the single-photon systems considered by Flower *et al.*, (1981) the gamma camera had the highest MSS if more than 10 sections were required.

An actual reconstruction of a uniformly filled cylinder is a crucial test of performance of systems in tomographic mode. Whilst resolution measurements are influenced by the reconstruction algorithm and provide vital information on the effectiveness of collimation, the effectiveness of attenuation correction can best be examined on a uniform distribution. Such a reconstruction also provides information on the effects of Poisson noise in real data. Any non-uniformity in sensitivity over the detector surface (gamma camera) or non-uniformity of sensitivity between discrete detectors will give rise to potentially severe artefacts in the reconstruction. Such non-uniformity should of course be fully investigated by conventional means (Section 5.6) and minimised before tomography is attempted. Likewise, the rigidity of the rotational mechanism and the alignment of the system (e.g., gamma camera axes) must also be fully investigated to ensure that the raw data are as consistent as possible with the assumed line integrals.

5.9   Choice of performance parameters

With such a wide range of parameters, the main problem facing a potential user is one of choice. To a great extent this choice will be limited by the specific requirements of the task in hand and whether subjective or objective measurements are preferred. Both of these considerations will be discussed later. Notwithstanding, if a parameter is to be of value it must satisfy the following four fundamental criteria.

(i)   Relevance. The purpose of the device is to image the distribution of radiopharmaceutical in a patient, so a parameter should relate to the conditions under which the device is to operate. For example, spatial resolution must be measured in a tissue-equivalent scattering medium rather than air. The discussion in Section 5.4 shows that temporal resolution should also be measured with scatter present.

This problem of relevance is brought out in the difference between the NEMA and IEC recommendations. NEMA recommendations are formulated by equipment manufacturers, so they place the emphasis on performance of the device *per se*, while the IEC proposals use more clinically realistic conditions. Undoubtedly the NEMA approach may be useful for the manufacturer as a quality control procedure, but performance figures which relate to clinical practice seem to be more appropriate for routine quality measurements.

(ii)   Simplicity. Regarding application to equipment in a hospital environment, the easier it is to make a measurement the more likely it is to be used. This is particularly true for regular quality control. Unfortunately the simplest measurements are rarely the most accurate. For example, FWHM of the LSF is often used to denote spatial resolution, but if the gamma rays being imaged have an energy which is slightly higher than that for which the collimator is designed, septal penetration can affect the tails of the LSF while leaving the FWHM unchanged.

(iii)   Sensitivity. It is not sufficient for a parameter to be relevant and simple to measure; it must also change significantly when there are clinically important variations in image quality. Unfortunately the sensitivity of a parameter is rarely known. For example, what change in the intrinsic resolution of a gamma camera represents a significant improvement in image quality? Differences as small as 0.5 mm (10%) are quoted in the manufacturer's literature as implying an improvement in performance. This is undoubtedly true in physical terms, but there is no experimental evidence to show that this change actually improves the clinical image.

Some work on this problem has been carried out by Kasal *et al.* (1983) on the sensitivity of FWHM as an indicator of image sharpness. They produced a set of gamma-camera images of a high-contrast edge taken at different spatial resolutions. Twelve observers were asked to rank these images in order of increasing sharpness. When at least nine observers agreed that one particular image was sharper than another, then, there is statistically significant evidence to reject the hypothesis that the images are indistinguishable. For FWHM values ranging from 5 mm to 2 cm, a 10% change in FWHM produced a perceptible change in sharpness.

To date this work has only been performed with the simplest of test patterns, but it demonstrates how the problem of measuring sensitivity may be approached.

(iv) Reproducibility. While the importance of sensitivity has been emphasised, it is equally important that sensitivity is not achieved at the expense of reproducibility.

5.9.1 Subjective versus objective tests

It is obvious that any assessment of imaging device performance should involve, at some stage, a visual examination of images, but such subjective tests are difficult to devise, particularly if one specific aspect of performance is to be investigated. For example, spatial resolution as measured by a quadrant bar phantom will depend not only upon device resolution but also upon the effectiveness of the display, image count density and the observer's visual judgement.

Objective measures, i.e., those not involving an observer, are often highly specific and reproducible yet they can be criticised as being isolated from the perceptual problem and so difficult to relate to image quality. For example, it is difficult to appreciate how image quality will be affected by a particular shape of transfer function. That said, there are certain aspects of device performance which can perhaps only be described in objective terms, in particular those describing the device's ability to produce accurate quantitative data, e.g., temporal resolution.

Frequently lacking is any knowledge about how objective measures relate to subjective tests. Sharp and Marshall (1981) looked for a correlation between certain objective measures of uniformity and subjective impression of uniformity. A set of flood images with varying degrees of non-uniformity was produced by varying the window width of the gamma camera's pulse height analyser. Six observers were then asked to rank the images in order of uniformity, and this subjective ranking was compared with the rankings produced when the images were arranged according to the values of the objective measures of uniformity. Four objective measures were tested, integral uniformity [(Eq. (5.15) and (5.16)], differential uniformity [Eq. (5.18)], coefficient of variation of the counts per pixel [Eq. (5.21)] and the spread of the differential uniformity [Eq. (5.22)]. Using Spearman's rank correlation coefficient to compare subjective and objective ordering, all four objective measures were found to agree well with the subjective impression of uniformity, the spread of differential uniformity showing closest agreement.

Kasal and Sharp (1985) have looked at the agreement between minimum discriminable bar separation and spatial resolution as measured by FWHM. Figure 5.8 shows that there is a linear relationship between the

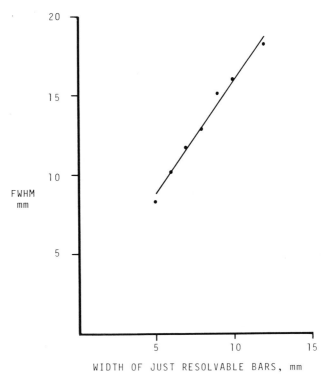

FIG. 5.8. Minimum resolvable bar width as a function of the spatial resolution (FWHM of the LSF) of the imaging system. [Figure provided by Mr. B. Kasal, University of Zagreb.]

two, so bar width and FWHM are assessing resolution in a similar way, but results depend upon image count density.

Subjective tests, although lacking specificity, have the advantage that they can test the complete imaging system. This so-called holistic approach to system testing contrasts with the reductionist one in which system components are examined separately. While the latter allows problem areas to be identified rapidly it is lengthy to implement, and since parameters generally interact, the measurement of them in isolation is of limited value in determining how the complete system will behave. For example, the sensitivity and resolution of a collimator are related, and we can ask "Is a better image produced by choosing high sensitivity but poor resolution or vice versa?" Various figures of merit have been proposed which combine sensitivity and resolution; Beck and Harper (1968) suggested that the product $(MTF)^2 \times S$, where S is the sensitivity, should be maximised. Other figures of merit have been proposed by Rollo (1977), Mulder (1978) and Nusynowitz and Benedetto (1979). In our view, attempts to specify system performance by a single parameter, whilst attractive, are unlikely to be fruitful.

Several subjective tests attempt to assess the performance of the complete imaging system by requiring the observer to identify the minimum discernible contrast change in a test pattern and then interpret this in terms of minimum perceptible "lesion" size or contrast. An example of such a pattern, the William's liver slice phantom (Rogers, 1976), is shown in Fig. 5.9. There is little evidence to show that such simple patterns constitute a comprehensive evaluation of device performance, although it has been suggested (Todd-Pokropek, 1983) that they may be useful as a test of one particular aspect of performance, namely "contrast resolution".

5.10 Use of performance parameters

As stated in Section 5.1 performance parameters are needed for two types of evaluation: for maintaining a regular check on the performance of an instrument (quality control) and for intercomparison of imaging devices.

5.10.1 Quality control

It cannot be overemphasised that quality control measurements must be simple and quick to perform if they are to be of any value. Daily measurements of certain parameters are important and in our experience need take no longer than 15 min to carry out. While they must be

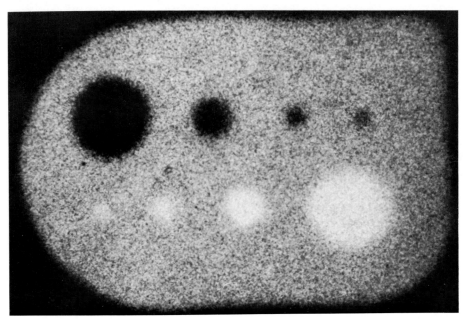

FIG. 5.9. Image of the Williams liver slice phantom. The diameters of the circular 'lesions' are 0.5, 1, 2 and 4 cm.

comprehensive, simplicity and sensitivity are more important than relevance.

The value of a simple measurement of performance is shown in Fig. 5.10. Daily measurements were made of the behaviour of the two detectors of a rectilinear scanner by placing a flood source of 133-Ba between the detectors and noting that setting of the pulse height analyser corresponding to the photo-peak. While the setting for the lower detector remained constant, that for the upper one fell steadily.

One major problem in quality control is deciding when there has been a significant deterioration in performance for remedial action to be necessary, i.e., defining the action threshold. The small but steady drop in the value of a measurement, as in Fig. 5.10, is much more difficult to detect than a sudden major fault such as caused by the failure of a PMT. Regular monitoring of device performance over an extended period allows us to assess the normal variability in the values of the chosen quality control parameters and to carry out standard statistical tests on a daily basis. While a cursory glance at a flood image may miss subtle changes, a computer analysis of uniformity parameters can be used to draw the operator's attention to the fact that these are statistically significant differences from normal.

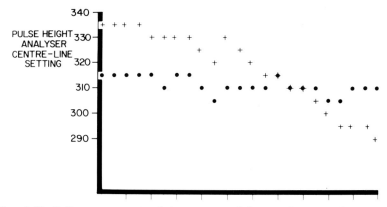

FIG. 5.10. Daily measurements of the response of the two detectors of a rectilinear scanner. Response was simply measured in terms of the pulse height analyser setting corresponding to the photo-peak of 133-Ba. The settings for the lower head (●) remain constant while those for the upper head (+) show a steady drop.

It is worth emphasising that since uniformity is affected by several factors, an abnormal flood image is non-specific as to the cause but it may prove a simple yet comprehensive quality control test. Figure 5.11 illustrates a typical quality control procedure based on the flood image together with daily and monthly computer print-out of the measurements.

Measurement of device performance is only one aspect of the quality control necessary in a nuclear medicine service; other parts of the imaging chain such as radiopharmaceutical quality must be taken into account. A more detailed consideration can be found in Rollo (1977) and Paras (1980).

5.10.2 Intercomparison of devices

In an intercomparison of imaging devices, the relevance and sensitivity of the measurements are more important than simplicity. It is not possible to specify precisely how measurements should be made as this will depend upon the type of device being examined, but the list of parameters given earlier is the minimum that should be considered.

Two points are perhaps worth making. First, the MTF is a most comprehensive measure of resolution and should be applied more widely. Its use does depend upon the imaging system being linear, but any system should be linear particularly if data is to be quantified. If the MTFs are not normalised they can be used to show relative sensitivity as well as spatial performance. Second, objective measurements of physical performance are only one part of the assessment of any device, and when devices of

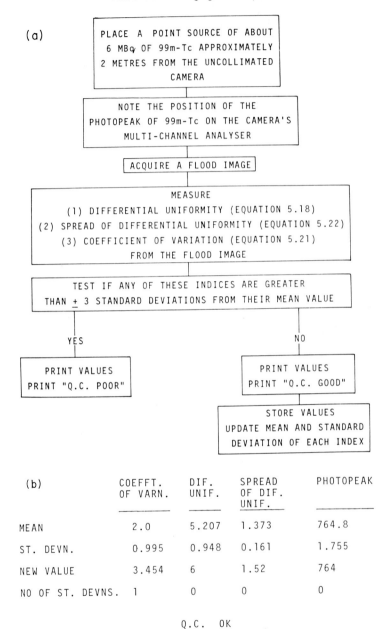

(a)

PLACE A POINT SOURCE OF ABOUT
6 MBq OF 99m-Tc APPROXIMATELY
2 METRES FROM THE UNCOLLIMATED
CAMERA

NOTE THE POSITION OF THE
PHOTOPEAK OF 99m-Tc ON THE CAMERA'S
MULTI-CHANNEL ANALYSER

ACQUIRE A FLOOD IMAGE

MEASURE
(1) DIFFERENTIAL UNIFORMITY (EQUATION 5.18)
(2) SPREAD OF DIFFERENTIAL UNIFORMITY (EQUATION 5.22)
(3) COEFFICIENT OF VARIATION (EQUATION 5.21)
FROM THE FLOOD IMAGE

TEST IF ANY OF THESE INDICES ARE GREATER
THAN $\pm$ 3 STANDARD DEVIATIONS FROM THEIR MEAN VALUE

YES   NO

PRINT VALUES   PRINT VALUES
PRINT "Q.C. POOR"   PRINT "Q.C. GOOD"

STORE VALUES
UPDATE MEAN AND STANDARD
DEVIATION OF EACH INDEX

(b)	COEFFT. OF VARN.	DIF. UNIF.	SPREAD OF DIF. UNIF.	PHOTOPEAK
MEAN	2.0	5.207	1.373	764.8
ST. DEVN.	0.995	0.948	0.161	1.755
NEW VALUE	3.454	6	1.52	764
NO OF ST. DEVNS.	1	0	0	0

Q.C. OK

FIG. 5.11. (a) Outline of a simple quality control routine for daily use. (b) Typical print-out of the results of a day's quality measurements. (c) Print-out of a month's measurements. The dashed lines show ± 3 standard deviations from the mean value of each index.

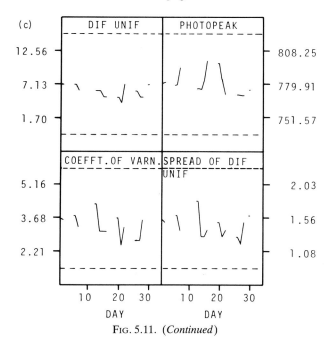

FIG. 5.11. (*Continued*)

fundamentally different modes of operation are being compared, e.g., a gamma camera and a tomographic scanner, it may be difficult to find common ground for comparison. Thus, ideally, any comparison should include clinical evaluation under controlled conditions. At the very least, 'typical' clinical images should be shown so that a reader may make his own judgement.

5.11   Concluding remarks

The publication of standards for quality measurements by NEMA, IEC and the HPA is an important first step for assessing the performance of imaging devices. It is unfortunate, however, that relatively little work has been published on the effectiveness of these performance indices for expressing image quality. There is still a gap between being able to specify certain features of imaging device performance and making measurements of parameters which are known to be very sensitive to changes in the quality of clinical images. For the former the standards are very effective but the latter are most relevant to the regular checks which should be made on clinical imaging equipment. This gap is perhaps, a result of the difficulty in linking the subjective impression of image quality with a quantitative measure which is required for an objective quality assurance procedure.

It cannot be overemphasised that to be effective quality assurance testing of a device must be made frequently. This, in turn, requires the tests to be simple and quick to perform. The NEMA, IEC and HPA standards are not designed for this purpose. The flood uniformity image probably provides the best, and certainly the simplest, general test pattern for daily use. It does, however, need to be supplemented with some form of test for spatial resolution.

With the development of more sophisticated imaging equipment the need for quality checks becomes greater. No doubt devices will be made self checking to a certain extent, but correction circuits, such as for linearity and energy, may conceal potentially serious faults, and the performance of equipment should be checked with the correction circuits switched off.

References

Adams, R., Jansen, C., Grames, M. and Zimmerman, C. D. (1974). Deadtime of scintillation camera systems—definitions, measurement and applications. *Med. Phys.* **1**, 198–203.

Adams, R., Hine, G. J. and Zimmerman, C. D. (1978). Deadtime measurements in scintillation cameras under scatter conditions simulating quantitative nuclear cardiography. *J. Nucl. Med.* **19**, 538–544.

Anger, H. O. (1973). Testing the performance of scintillation cameras. *Lawrence Berkeley Lab.* [*Rep.*] *LBL* **LBL-2027.**

Beck, R. N. and Harper, P. V. (1968). Criteria for evaluating radioisotope imaging systems. *In* "Fundamental Problems in Scanning", (A. Gottschalk and R. N. Beck, eds.), pp. 348–384. Charles C. Thomas, Springfield, Illinios.

Causer, D. A. and Mallard, J. R. (1974). Measurement of the sensitivity of gamma ray imaging systems. *Int. J. Appl. Radiat. Isot.* **25**, 119–129.

Cox, N. J. and Diffey, B. L. (1976). A numerical index of gamma-camera uniformity. *Br. J. Radiol.* **49**, 734–735.

Evans, R. D. (1955). "The Atomic Nucleus", pp. 785–788. McGraw-Hill, New York.

Flower, M. A., Rowe, R. W., Webb, S. and Keyes, W. I. (1981). A comparison of three systems for performing single-photon emission tomography. *Phys. Med. Biol.* **26**, 671–691.

Guldberg, C. and Rossing, N. (1978). Comparing the performance of two gamma-cameras under high counting rates: principles and practice. *J. Nucl. Med.* **19**, 545–552.

Hine, G. J., Paras, P. and Warr, C. P. (1977). Measurements of the performance parameters of gamma-cameras: Part 1. *DHEW Publ. (FDA) (U.S.)* **FDA-78–8049.**

Hine, G. J., Paras, P., Warr, C. P. and Adams, R. (1979). Measurements of the performance parameters of gamma-cameras: Part II. **DHEW Publ.** *(FDA) (U.S.)* **FDA–79–8049.**

Horton, P. W., Leach, K. G., Griffiths, J. T., Hawkins, L. A., O'Hewell, D., Short, M. D., Todd, J. H., Turner, P. C. R., Wilks, R. J. and Murray, K. J. (1978). "The Theory, Specification and Testing of Anger Type Gamma-Cameras", Topic Group Report 27. The Hospital Physicists' Association, London.

Kasal, B. and Sharp, P. F. (1985). Gamma camera spatial resolution as measured by the bar phantom. *Phys. Med. Biol.* **30**, 263–266.

Kasal, B., Sharp, P. F. and Dendy, P. P. (1983). Relationship between objective and subjective assessment of gamma-camera image sharpness. *Phys. Med. Biol.* **28**, 1127–1134.

MacIntyre, W. A., Fedoruk, S. O., Harris, C. C., Kuhl, D. E. and Mallard, J. R. (1969). Sensitivity and resolution in radioisotope scanning. *In* "Medical Radioisotope Scintigraphy", Vol. 1, pp. 391–434. IAEA, Vienna.

Muehllehner, G. and Colsher, J. G. (1983). Scintillation camera. *In* "Principles of Radionuclide Emission Imaging" (D. E. Kuhl, ed.), pp. 1–25. Pergamon Press, New York.

Muehllehner, G., Colsher, J. G. and Stoub, E. W. (1980). Correction for non-uniformity in scintillation cameras through removal of spatial distortion. *J. Nucl. Med.* **21**, 771–776.

Muehllehner, G., Wake, R. H. and Sano, R. (1981). Standards for performance measurements in scintillation cameras. *J. Nucl. Med.* **22**, 72–77.

Mulder, H. (1978). Definition of a quality factor for medical scintillation cameras. *Oldelft Sci. Eng. Q.* **1**, 17–26.

Murphy, P., Arsenau, R., Maxon, E. and Thompson, W. (1977). Clinical significance of scintillation camera electronics capable of high processing rates. *J. Nucl. Med.* **18**, 175–179.

Nusynowitz, M. L. and Benedetto, A. R. (1979). A mathematical index of uniformity (IOU) for sensitivity and resolution. *Radiology* **131**, 235–241.

Paras, P. (1976). Quality assurance in nuclear medicine. *In* "Medical Radionuclide Imaging", pp. 3–39. IAEA, Vienna.

Paras, P. (1980). Performance and quality control of nuclear medicine instrumentation. *In* "Medical Radionuclide Imaging", pp. 79–140. IAEA, Vienna.

Rogers, T. T. (1976). A survey of images of a phantom produced by radioisotope scanners and cameras. *Spec. Rep.—Br. Inst. Radiol.* No. 9.

Rollo, F. D. (1977). Evaluating imaging devices. *In* "Nuclear Medicine Physics, Instrumentation and Agents" (F. D. Rollo, ed.), Chap. 11. C. V. Mosby, St. Louis, Missouri.

Ross. D. A. and Harris, C. C. (1969). Measurement of radioactivity. *In* "Principles of Nuclear Medicine" (H. N. Wagner, ed.), pp. 130–258. W. B. Saunders, Philadelphia, Pennsylvania.

Sano, R. M. (1980). Performance standards. *In* "Medical Radionuclide Imaging", Vol. 2, pp. 141–159. IAEA, Vienna.

Sharp, P. and Marshall, I. (1981). The usefulness of indices measuring gamma-camera non-uniformity. *Phys. Med. Biol.* **26**, 149–153.

Strand, S. E. and Larsson, I. (1978). Image artifacts at high photon fluence rates in single-crystal NaI(Tl) scintillation cameras. *J. Nucl. Med.* **19**, 407–413.

Todd-Pokropek, A. (1983). Quality control, detection and display. *In* "Principles of Radionuclide Emission Imaging" (D. E. Kuhl, ed.), pp. 27–76. Pergamon Press, New York.

Van Tuinen, R. J., Kruger, J. B., Bahr, G. K. and Sodd, V. J. (1978). Scintillation camera non-uniformity: effects on cold lesion detectability. *Int. J. Nucl.Med. Biol.* **5**, 135–140.

Chapter 6

Other Imaging Devices

6.1 Introduction

It is evident from Chapter 3 that both the gamma camera and rectilinear scanner have limited imaging capabilities. Several other devices have been proposed, although it must be stated that, except for certain very specialised investigations, the gamma camera still remains the instrument of choice.

Three categories of imaging devices will be considered in this chapter. The first consists of those using the conventional NaI(Tl) scintillation detector, in one case in conjunction with an image intensifier to improve photon statistics, in a second as a multi-crystal configuration to simplify the pulse arithmetic circuits and, finally, in the hybrid scanner.

The second category encompasses devices using detectors other than the scintillation crystal, namely the gas-filled multi-wire proportional counter and the solid-state detector.

In all of these devices a collimator must be used to image radionuclides emitting single gamma rays, and, consequently, sensitivity is severely reduced. The third category represents those devices which do not require a collimator, the Compton-effect camera and coded aperture detectors.

6.2   Devices based on the NaI(TI) scintillation detector

6.2.1   The intensifier camera

Many of the imaging problems of the gamma camera derive from the fairly low number of light photons, approximately 4000 from a 140-keV 99m-Tc gamma ray, which are shared between as many as 91 PMTs. Using an image intensifier and electron multiplier, a photon gain in excess of 10,000 can be achieved. Originally it was suggested that an X-ray amplifier could be used (Kellershohn and Pellerin, 1955). However, such a device is an inefficient gamma-ray detector, even at 99m-Tc energies, and it was necessary to use a conventional NaI(Tl) crystal coupled to the photo-cathode of the intensifier (see, e.g., Mitchell *et al.*, 1973; Mulder and Pauwels, 1976). As with a gamma camera, the gamma ray flux must first be collimated to produce an image in the detector.

While it is possible to photograph the intensified image on the output screen directly, pulse height analysis and data quantification are more easily performed if the amplified image is converted into electronic signals and then redisplayed. Roux *et al.* (1972) have shown that for the minified image produced by an intensifier, four PMTs are sufficient to calculate accurately the spatial coordinates of the intense output signals.

In a camera described by Driard *et al.* (1971) (Fig. 6.1), a single collimated NaI(Tl) scintillation crystal is connected directly to the photo-cathode of a cascaded two-stage image intensifier, the second stage incorporating an electron multiplier. The 2-cm-diameter output screen is viewed by four PMTs (3.2 cm in diameter) whose signals feed circuits producing conventional X, Y and Z (energy) pulses. As the photon gain varies over the face of the output screen, a compensating filter is placed

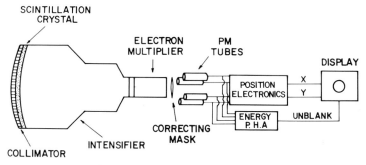

Fig. 6.1. Intensifier gamma camera.

between it and the PMTs. In a commercial version of this device a 32-cm field of view was achieved with an intrinsic resolution of 4.5 mm FWHM at 140 keV. A maximum count rate of 100 kcps was claimed.

6.2.2 Multi-crystal detectors

The use of a single large scintillation crystal as a gamma-ray detector with analogue position calculation also has the disadvantage of loss of sensitivity at high energies resulting from the need to use a thin crystal. If the single crystal is replaced by a mosaic of small crystals isolated from each other, the position of an event can be calculated simply by recording the crystal in which the event occurred. Electronic pulse analysis can be faster since the need for summed weighted signals and ratio circuits is removed thus giving improved high count rate performance. Sensitivity at higher energies is also increased since there is no limitation on maximum crystal thickness.

Multi-crystal detectors were first suggested by Bender and Blau (1963) almost simultaneously with the Anger camera but have never achieved the latter's popularity. One commercial system with a detector made up of 294 NaI(Tl) crystals each $\frac{5}{16}$ in. square and 1.5 in. thick is available. Each crystal has a separate can optically isolating it from the others, and a system of light guides is used to direct the signals from the crystals to an array of 35 2-in. PMTs in such a way that each crystal is uniquely addressed by a pair of PMTs, one identifying its X coordinate, the other its Y coordinate (Fig. 6.2). When used in high count rate studies, the position signals are sent directly to a computer memory store after conventional pulse height analysis. Collimation is still required, but in this digital system it is obviously sufficient to have one collimator hole per crystal. Tapered holes are used and resolution depends on hole length.

The major advantage of this device is its ability to handle high count rates. Since pulse mixing is not necessary to give photon location, the greatest delay in pulse processing is writing into the device's memory store. Little distortion is evident up to count rates of 100 kcps and the maximum recorded count rate is as high as 400 kcps. The multi-crystal detector has, as a consequence, been found to be of greatest value in "first pass" cardiac imaging.

A second point in favour of the multi-crystal detector is that the 1.5-in.-thick crystals give higher sensitivity to high-energy gamma rays than the gamma camera (see Fig. 3.12).

Since the spatial location of a detected gamma ray is known only to within the dimensions of a single crystal, intrinsic resolution is worse than in a conventional gamma camera. This problem is overcome in static

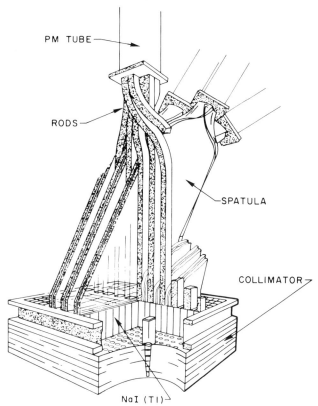

FIG. 6.2. Cut-away diagram of the multi-crystal detector. (Courtesy of the Baird Corporation.)

studies by moving the patient's couch over a 4 × 4 matrix, each step being one quarter of the inter-crystal spacing. Obviously this technique cannot be used during dynamic studies.

A second problem is that, as 24-in.-long light guides are used to connect PMTs to the crystals, there is appreciable light loss and degradation of the energy signal. In practice the energy resolution is only about 50%. To compensate for this a certain amount of scatter is removed by filters positioned in front of the crystal assembly.

6.2.3 Hybrid scanners

In a hybrid scanner a long narrow bar of NaI(Tl) or a linear array of smaller crystals is used as the detector, the position of an event along the long axis of the crystal normally being measured by an array of PMTs. The orthogonal coordinate is found from the position of the detector as it moves in a direction perpendicular to the crystal axis. Coordinate computation is therefore a combination of that used in the gamma camera and that used in the rectilinear scanner.

These devices are useful for whole-body imaging since, if the detector is long enough to cover the width of the body, a single pass along the length of the body suffices. Since the PMT signals are only used to calculate one coordinate, the NaI(Tl) crystal may be thicker than that in a gamma camera, thus giving better sensitivity for higher-energy gamma rays.

In one commercial version of this device, a linear array of six PMTs views a 2-cm-thick, 50-cm-long crystal, and event position in the crystal is determined using arithmetic similar to that of the gamma camera. Another type of hybrid scanner uses a linear array of individual crystals, each with its own PMT and collimator hole.

A third type uses only two PMTs, one at each end of the crystal looking along its length (Davis and Martonne, 1966). If V_1 and V_2 are the signals from each PMT produced by a single scintillation, then, assuming simple linear attenuation of the light flash along the crystal, it can be shown that $(V_1 V_2)^{1/2}$ is proportional to the gamma-ray energy and $\log V_1/V_2$ to the position of the scintillation.

6.3   Devices not using the scintillation detector

6.3.1   The semi-conductor camera

In a conventional gamma camera the energy resolution is about 12% at 140 keV, so to ensure that a high proportion of the photo-peak events are imaged, a 20–30% energy window must be used on the pulse height analyser. Unfortunately, at low photon energies the change in energy resulting from Compton scattering is small and the scattered photon is likely to be accepted within the analyser window. For 140-keV 99m-Tc gamma rays, a 20% window with a lower energy level set at 126 keV only discriminates effectively against gamma rays scattered through more than 45°, so typically 30% of the photons forming the final image have been scattered. This poor energy resolution arises because about 300 eV of energy must be deposited in an NaI(Tl) detector to produce one electron at the PMT photocathode. On the other hand, in a high purity germanium detector only 2.9 eV is needed to produce one electron–hole pair; thus one 140-keV gamma ray will produce about 50,000 electrons. The statistical fluctuation associated with this signal is much lower so energy resolution of the order of 1% may be achieved. Discrimination against scatter is then effective even at low energies.

Initially, solid-state detector imaging devices employed lithium-drifted silicon or germanium detectors (Parker *et al.*, 1973) which had to be kept cool to maintain the doping. Detectors using high purity $(10^9–10^{11}$ electrical impurities/cm^3) germanium are now available and only require cooling during operation to minimise thermally induced noise.

The development of semi-conductor gamma cameras has also been limited by the small crystal areas available, with the largest used to date in a camera having a 6.4×3.2 cm^2 surface made from two 1-cm-thick crystals (Kaufman *et al.*, 1978) although crystals are available with uniform areas of 5×15 cm^2.

Positional information is obtained by using an orthogonal strip read-out. This involves cutting sets of parallel grooves in the *n* and *p* sides, one set orthogonal to the other, to produce electrically isolated strips of detector (Fig. 6.3). In one camera (Kaufman *et al.*, 1978) the *n* side consists of lithium diffused into germanium with grooves 0.5 mm wide and 2 mm pitch cut through the lithium layer. The *p* surface is made of palladium over germanium oxide, the groove width being 200 μm and again 2 mm pitch. The device thus acts, in theory, as an array of 2-mm-square detectors, and so by attaching electrodes to the top and bottom surfaces of each detector element, the spatial position of an event can be determined. This gives very good intrinsic spatial resolution, with a theoretically rectangular point spread function (PSF) of full width 2 mm. In practice the spatial resolution

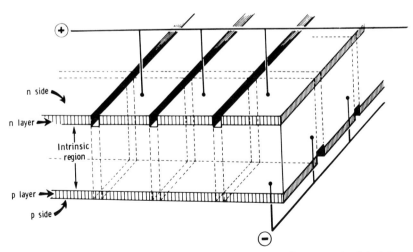

Fig. 6.3. Detector array for a semi-conductor camera. [From Detko (1969).]

is limited by reduced photo-peak efficiency, scatter and an increase in edge of field effect which accompanies decreasing element size.

Such an instrument still requires collimation to produce an image on the detector array, and, as with any multi-detector device, each detector element should have its own collimator channel. Because of the excellent energy resolution, it is not necessary for the septa to stop obliquely incident gamma rays, but simply to scatter them sufficiently for discrimination to occur in the pulse height analysis circuits. Thus, septa walls can be thin even at quite high energies.

Since event detection is only a matter of charge collection from a detector element, performance at high count rates is solely limited by pulse processing times and even in the prototype devices is very fast. Table 6.1 shows typical performance characteristics.

Other promising semi-conductor detector materials include cadmium telluride and sulphide, gallium arsenide and phosphide, lead iodide and oxide and mercuric oxide. However, if they are to be stable in a clinical environment, then high manufacturing standards are needed.

6.3.2   The multi-wire proportional chamber

The multi-wire proportional chamber (MWPC) was originally designed for high-energy physics experiments. It consists of a gas-filled chamber containing three planes of wires, the central anode plane being kept at a positive potential with respect to the two outer cathode planes. The wires of one cathode are orthogonal to those of the other. Any ionization in the gas produces free electrons which are attracted to an anode wire where an electron avalanche is generated on the high electric field. Signals induced

TABLE 6.1. Performance of a prototype semi-conductor gamma camera.

Spatial resolution	2 mm[a]
	5 mm[b]
Maximum count rate	250 kcps
Sensitivity	14×10^{-4} cps/Bq[c]
Energy resolution	3%[d]
Detector area	64×32 mm^2

[a] Intrinsic resolution.
[b] At 10 cm depth in tissue using a high resolution collimator.
[c] With a high resolution collimator.
[d] At 140 keV.

in the several cathode wires centred on the avalanche position can be used to compute the X and Y coordinates of the avalanche (Fig. 6.4). As an imaging device for gamma rays it suffers from the obvious difficulty of stopping the photons in the gas filling of the chamber. Photoelectric converters have been used to improve sensitivity and can be situated either inside the chamber or between the chamber and patient.

An MWPC using internal converters was constructed for single-photon imaging by Bateman and Connolly (1978). The converter, which consisted of tin attached to a plastic support, also acted as the cathode. The tin was divided into strips, those in adjacent cathode planes running orthogonally. Between the cathodes was a plane of anode wires of 20 μm diameter (Fig. 6.5.). An incident gamma photon undergoes photoelectric absorption in the tin releasing a shower of photoelectrons into the chamber. Obviously the tin foil must be sufficiently thin to allow these electrons to escape, and consequently its ability to stop the gamma photons is reduced. Even though the gas in the chamber will stop all the photoelectrons, the overall detection efficiency of one chamber is only about 1% and several chambers must be stacked to achieve a reasonable efficiency. In Bateman's device 25 layers were used, giving an efficiency of about 15% for 140-keV gamma rays.

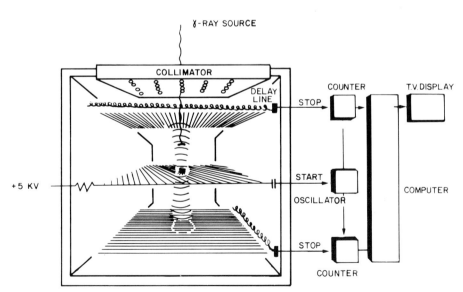

FIG. 6.4. The basic multi-wire proportional chamber as an imaging device.

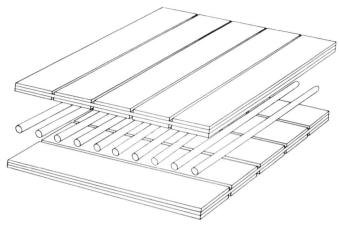

FIG. 6.5. Internal converters for MWPCs as proposed by Bateman and Connolly. [From Bateman and Connolly (1978).]

The electrons are attracted to the nearest anode wire, generating an electron avalanche in the high electric field, so inducing charge signals on both the anode wire and the two nearest cathodes. The cathode strips conduct the signal to two delay line readout systems which permit measurement of the event's X and Y coordinates (Reading, 1976). The Z coordinate (depth) of interaction is measured from the anode plane signal and is used to correct for parallax effects in the thick detector.

To achieve good spatial resolution, the lateral spread of the photoelectrons must be minimised by making the cathode–anode gap as small as possible and by using a dense gas as the chamber filling. Using a 5-mm cathode–anode separation and a filling of pressurised isobutane, lead bars 1.6 mm wide were imaged with 120-keV gamma rays.

The preceding measurement refers to the intrinsic resolution of the chamber, and in clinical practice it is necessary to use a conventional collimator. The 15% detection efficiency, prior to collimation, compares unfavourably with the 95% efficiency of the gamma camera detector. Even the possible advantage of being able to manufacture very large area detectors seems unlikely to offset this disadvantage.

More recently, the MWPC has been used for positron imaging, a pair of detectors forming a coincidence imaging system (see Section 4.5). To deal with the higher-energy gamma rays produced by positron annihilation, lead converters are used instead of tin foil. Figure 6.6 shows such a system having 21 cathode planes and a detector area of 30×30 cm^2 (Bateman) et $al.$, 1983). The sensitivity of this system is about 0.05% and spatial resolution is 6 mm full width at half-maximum height (FWHM).

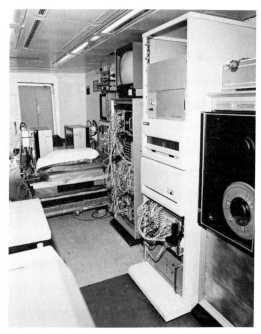

FIG. 6.6. An MWPC system used for coincidence imaging. The two detectors are in the background behind the couch, with the nucleonics and computer system in the foreground. [Photograph courtesy of Dr. J. E. Bateman, Rutherford Laboratory, Chilton, Oxfordshire.]

The external gamma ray converter (Jeavons *et al.*, 1975; Chu *et al.*, 1977) consists of matrix of holes in a lead sheet. An electric field is applied across the converter so that electrons resulting from an interaction of the gamma ray within the lead are drifted out of the converter along the holes and into the detector chambers (Fig. 6.7). At 140 keV, the range of the photoelectron is so short that 0.08-mm-diameter holes and 0.1-mm centres would be needed, with consequent fabrication problems. However, at positron annihilation radiation energies such a converter is feasible, hole diameters of 0.8 mm with a pitch of 1 mm being a typical requirement, and detection efficiencies of about 30% are claimed to be possible. At present the overall sensitivity of the device is about 0.3%.

When an external converter is used, the problem of spatial degradation by long-range electrons is reduced since the primary high energy photoelectron or Compton electron that escapes from the wall of the converter interacts with the gas in the channels to produce the free electrons which are then drifted into the chamber. This gives a spatial resolution of 2–3 mm.

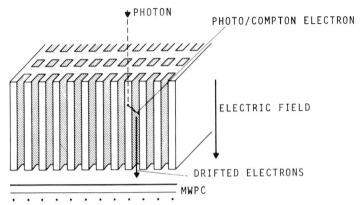

FIG. 6.7. External gamma ray converter for an MWPC. [From Jeavons *et al.* (1978). Copyright © 1978 IEEE.]

6.4 Devices not using collimators

6.4.1 Compton-effect camera

The theory of Compton scattering gives a unique relationship between the fractional energy loss in the interaction and the angle through which the gamma ray is scattered. So by assuming that photons arriving at the camera carry the full photo-peak energy, precise measurement of both the energy lost when a gamma photon is first Compton scattered in the detector and its subsequent trajectory permits its point of origin to be calculated. In Fig.6.8 a photon interacts with the detector at A and B. By measuring the energy lost at A, the scatter angle θ can be calculated. The point of emission of the gamma ray is then known to lie on the surface of the cone of semi-angle θ whose axis is the post-scatter trajectory AB extrapolated back towards the patient (the broken line in Fig. 6.8). Given several gamma rays emitted from the same place, the point of intersection of their respective cones is the origin of the photons. Thus, it is possible, in theory, to produce a three-dimensional image of the radionuclide distribution without the aid of a collimator.

Several requirements must first be met, however. The accuracy with which the energy deposited at A is measured must be very high as it will ultimately determine spatial resolution. Only a semi-conductor detector will have sufficiently good energy resolution.

Secondly, in order to discriminate against photons which have been scattered in the patient, it is necessary to know the energy of the photons incident on the detector. This can be done by assuming that all energy is

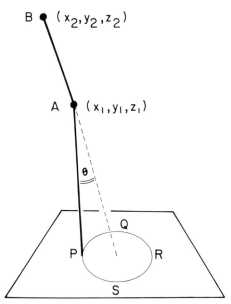

FIG. 6.8. Trajectory of a gamma ray which is Compton scattered at A and B in the detector. The computed origin of the gamma ray is on the surface of the cone of angle θ, which intersects the plane at PQRS.

lost in the first two interactions, a reasonable assumption for photons of about 100 keV, and measuring energy loss at both A and B. Alternatively by recording the position of the first three interactions together with the energy loss at the first two, the energy of the incident photon can be measured precisely. Finally, the detector sensitivity depends upon its area and source–detector distance.

Two designs for this device have been proposed. The first consists of a three-dimensional array of silicon detectors (Todd *et al.*, 1974; Everett *et al.*, 1976). Its performance has only been tested by computer simulation, a point source of 1.25-MeV photons being imaged with a spatial resolution of 5 mm. The PSF, however, had a long tail. Its size was significant 6 mm from the peak and this will degrade image quality. To date no working version of this device has been built.

The second version of the Compton-effect camera uses a hybrid detector. This consists of a semi-conductor detector made of germanium behind which is a second detector, an uncollimated gamma camera (Singh, 1983; Singh and Doria, 1983). A prototype device has been built using a 33×33 array of $5 \times 5 \text{ mm}^2$ cryogenically cooled germanium detectors. Spatial resolution of less than 1.2 mm is claimed with a sensitivity for 140-keV gamma photons about 15 times higher than that of a conventional gamma camera. Unfortunately, the potential of this high sensitivity cannot be realised as the gamma camera part of the detector is inadequate in dealing with the resulting high count rates.

The major problem with the Compton-effect camera, yet to be resolved, is whether it is possible to reconstruct the image with sufficient accuracy and sufficiently quickly to make full three-dimensional clinical imaging feasible.

6.4.2   Coded aperture imaging

The idea of replacing the conventional collimater by a coded aperture was first suggested by Barrett (1972). This aperture is made up of areas transparent and opaque to gamma rays. When it is inserted between the patient and a suitable detector, shadows of the aperture are thrown onto the detector, each point source of radioactivity in the patient producing its own shadow.

The location of the shadow on the detector is determined by the position of the gamma-ray source in the plane parallel to the detector while the magnification of the aperture image depends upon the distance of the source from the aperture (Fig. 6.9). The intensity of the source will be reflected in the density of the aperture image.

To form the final image this coded data must be decoded. This can be done by correlating a 'mask' of the same form as the aperture with the coded image. Those positions at which the mask matches an aperture shadow correspond to the spatial locations of gamma-ray point sources, and the total of all such point sources constitutes the decoded image. By altering the size of the mask, images of different planes in the patient can be reconstructed. It must be noted, however, that not all coded aperture systems are capable of tomography.

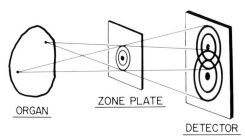

ORGAN

ZONE PLATE

DETECTOR

FIG. 6.9. Production of a coded image. The more distant of the two sources produces the smaller shadow of the zone plate on the detector. The lateral displacement of the two shadows is proportional to that of the two sources in the organ.

This process of correlating a mask with the coded image can be carried out either optically, by measuring the amount of light transmitted as a transparency of the mask is moved over a transparency of the coded image, or with a digital computer.

The effectiveness of an aperture depends upon it giving a unique coding for the spatial coordinates of the gamma-ray source. Any ambiguity as to the object distribution which produced a particular coded image is equivalent to a degradation of spatial resolution. A point source of activity will produce a coded image consisting of a single image of the aperture. By correlating the aperture mask with this image, the equivalent to the PSF of the aperture can be measured. The ideal aperture for coding would be one in which this auto-correlation function is sharply peaked, i.e., there is a strong signal when the mask is aligned precisely with its image, but no signal when the two are out of alignment.

The Fresnel zone plate was the first coded aperture to be used for medical imaging. It consists of a set of concentric annuli of equal area alternatively transparent and opaque to gamma rays (Fig. 6.10a). Since about half of the incident gamma rays will be transmitted, it will have a sensitivity several hundred times higher than the parallel-hole collimator.

The Fresnel zone plate has one important advantage over other types of coded aperture at the decoding stage. If the coded image is recorded as a transparency and a coherent light beam is shone through it (Fig. 6.11), each individual zone plate image will diffract the light to form a spot in the decoded image. The principal focal point of a zone plate depends upon the magnification of the zone plate which, as already mentioned, is determined by the distance of the gamma-ray source from the zone plate. So by moving the decoded image detector along the axis of the light beam different object planes can be brought into focus.

While the coded aperture imaging system has the disadvantage of needing a decoding stage, the advantage of high sensitivity plus the ability to reconstruct selected planes appears very attractive. Unfortunately there are several problems that make the simple zone plate unsuitable for clinical imaging.

The zone plate focuses the coherent light beam by diffraction, but there are several weaker focal spots in addition to the principal one, the focal lengths being r_1^2/nx where r_1 is the radius of the first annulus, x the wavelength of the coherent light, and $n = 0, \pm1, \pm3$, etc. Positive values of n correspond to virtual focal spots and negative values to real ones. Since a set of images is produced in different planes, there will be interference, particularly between the first-order real and first-order virtual images. Also there is an undiffracted component, corresponding to $n = 0$, making up 50% of the transmitted light. This will expose the decoded image

(a)

(b)

(c)

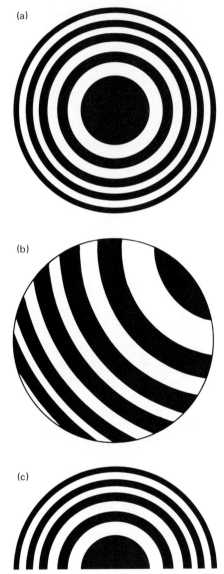

F_{IG}. 6.10. (a) Fresnel zone plate, (b) off-axis Fresnel zone plate and (c) single side-band zone plate.

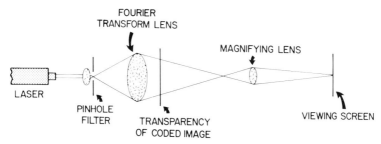

FIG. 6.11. Reconstruction of a coded image using coherent light.

uniformly, thereby lowering the contrast. Several methods have been used to reduce these effects, but they do so only at the expense of degrading the decoded image signal to noise ratio.

One interesting alternative approach is to use an off-axis zone plate (Fig. 6.10b), which allows the various diffracted orders n to be physically separated (Barrett *et al.*, 1972). Unfortunately, it only reproduces the high frequencies of the object, and so the object must first be modulated (heterodyned) with a high-frequency periodic grating. This immediately results in a 50% loss of emitted photons, of course, but it has been used in clinical practice. Crippin (1976) proposed that the so-called single side band zone plate (Fig. 6.10c) offered a way of separating out the different diffracted orders without needing to heterodyne the object. The optical reconstruction process with coherent light is not a satisfactory method in this case, and a digital correlation technique must be used.

One of the advantages of coded aperture imaging is high sensitivity, but at present it is difficult to find a suitable detector system for recording the coded image, most conventional imagers, such as the gamma camera, being unable to handle this high count rate. One attractive possibility is to use X-ray film together with intensifying screens to give a cheap and simple imaging system. This will, of course, result in a loss of sensitivity.

Surprisingly for an imaging system of such high sensitivity, achieving a high signal to noise ratio (SNR) is a problem. This is mainly because the spatial distribution of noise in the coded image is different from that in the conventional gamma-camera image. The difficulty arises in the decoding stage where every element in the coded image will contribute to every element in the decoded image so that the quantum noise is nearly constant over the decoded image. In areas of low count density the SNR will actually be lower than in a conventional image, but the reverse holds true in high count density regions. To this quantum noise must be added noise arising from the source distribution, noise introduced by the method of decoding and artefacts caused by the presence of incomplete projections of the zone plate onto the detector.

If the object is considered as consisting of M resolution areas, i.e., M point sources, then the SNR is (Barrett and De Meester, 1974)

$$\mathrm{SNR} = K\sqrt{N}/M \qquad (6.1)$$

where N is the total number of photons in the coded image and K a constant, of value between 0 and 1, which depends upon the method of decoding.

A point source is equivalent to the smallest resolvable detail in the object, so the spatial resolution of the zone plate will be determined by the ratio of object size to M. High spatial resolution can thus only be achieved when imaging small organs.

Coded apertures other than the variants on the zone plate have been used. Of particular interest are the multiple pinhole apertures with up to a hundred pinholes in a gamma-ray opaque sheet arranged in a so-called non-redundant pattern (see, e.g., Chang *et al.*, 1974) in which no repetition of hole pattern occurs. The auto-correlation function will thus show a maximum when complete alignment is achieved but otherwise no more than one pair of pinholes will be aligned. The coherent optical method of decoding is far more complicated than with the zone plate because of the need to generate a holographic spatial filter to perform cross-correlation. Digital processing, however, is comparable to that for zone plates. A consideration of the area of the aperture transparent to gamma photons will indicate that pinhole apertures are much less sensitive than zone plates.

The apertures considered so far are stationary, the configuration of transparent and opaque regions remaining unchanged during an exposure. Several workers have investigated the possibilities of time-dependent apertures. Koral and colleagues (1975), for example, used a pseudoran-dom coded pinhole plate to take a sequence of images, each one being pro-duced with a different arrangement of the pinholes. When this is used in conjunction with a simple detector to record the net photon flux through the aperture, a two-dimensional image can be reconstructed by back-projection of the signals through the pinholes. When the plate is used in conjunction with a detector system capable of giving the spatial distribu-tion of the incoming photon flux, such as a gamma camera, tomographic images can be reconstructed.

Macovski (1974) also used a multi-pinhole aperture but in a manner which allowed the image formed by each pinhole to be identified sepa-rately. This was achieved by modulating the transmission of each pinhole, using shutters opaque to gamma rays, at a characteristic frequency. The final image was reconstructed by first correcting for the angle from which each pinhole viewed the patient by shifting the X and Y coordinates of the pinhole's image so as to bring each image into alignment and then summing all images. As with any pinhole collimator, data from different planes in the patient will be imaged at a different magnification and this allows tomographic reconstruction to be carried out.

Keyes (1975) proposed that collimator sensitivity could be improved by constructing the collimator from an array of parallel slits rather than holes. As it is now not possible to discriminate spatially between photons incident through the same slit, an image will simply be a one-dimensional count density profile running perpendicular to the direction of the slits. To produce an image, a series of profiles is acquired as the collimator is rotated about its central axis, one profile for each orientation. By using a standard tomographic reconstruction algorithm (Section 4.4) these profiles can be reconstructed to give a conventional two-dimensional image.

Coded aperture imaging can thus be seen to encompass a wide variety of techniques. For a fuller description the reader is referred to the excellent account by Barrett and Swindell (1981). It must be said, however, that although the potential advantages are great, to date coded apertures have not found any significant role in routine clinical imaging.

6.5 Concluding remarks

While several ingenious proposals have been put forward for imaging radiopharmaceuticals, none has, so far, challenged the supremacy of the gamma camera.

One of the major difficulties in realising an improvement in image quality is that this will only result from improving one specific aspect of imaging device performance provided that others remain as good as for the camera. For example, we would undoubtedly like a device which has better spatial resolution than the 1–2 cm found in practice with the gamma camera. A significant improvement can only be achieved in clinical studies if this is coupled with good energy resolution and sensitivity. The former is necessary to exclude scattered radiation which would otherwise degrade significantly the resolution achieved without scatter present.

The importance of high sensitivity can be seen from the simple model of Chapter 2. Fine detail will be seen only if the SNR is sufficiently high. Since we are using a smaller acceptance cone, the number of counts in this area will be reduced, and hence the SNR lowered, unless the image count density is increased. For example, an increase in resolution of a factor of 10 will need a hundredfold increase in count density. Also, movement by the patient must now be minimised and short exposure times will be necessary.

The ideal imaging device would not only have much higher sensitivity than can be achieved by using a collimator but would also need to intercept a higher proportion of the emitted gamma rays. This latter requirement could only be met by a detector system which surrounded the patient. Multi-detector positron imagers (Section 4.5) probably come closest to this ideal device, but they do require a convenient source of positron-emitting radionuclides either from a nearby cyclotron or perhaps from a generator.

Coded aperture systems have their own limitations, the Fresnel zone plate being limited to small organs if high resolution is required, and a suitable detector has yet to be found. The semi-conductor detector is probably the most promising one and has excellent energy resolution, but at the present a large area device would be very expensive to build.

The Compton-effect camera too is limited by the availability of a suitable detector, but also there must be doubts as to whether the image reconstruction process can be implemented without very large computing resources.

While existing technology does not offer the potential for realising our ideal imaging device, there is still a useful role for some of these other devices in more specialised imaging tasks. The value of the multi-crystal detector for high count rate cardiac studies has already been mentioned, and a version of the hybrid scanner (Crawley *et al.*, 1981) has been adapted as a very simple imaging device for use in Third World countries.

References

Barrett, H. H. (1972). Fresnel zone plate imaging in nuclear medicine. *J. Nucl. Med.* **13,** 382–385.

Barrett, H. H. and De Meester, G. D. (1974). Quantum noise in Fresnel zone plate imaging. *Appl. Opt.* **13,** 1100–1109.

Barrett, H. H. and Swindell, W. (1981). "Radiological Imaging. The Theory of Image Formation, Detection and Processing", Vol. II, Chap. 8. Academic Press, New York and London.

Barrett, H. H., De Meester, G. D., Wilson, D. T. and Farmelant, M. H. (1972). Recent advances in Fresnel zone plate imaging. *In* "Medical Radioisotope Scintigraphy", Vol. 1, pp. 269–281. IAEA, Vienna.

Bateman, J. E. and Connolly, J. F. (1978). A multiwire proportional gamma-camera for imaging 99m-Tc radionuclide distributions. *Phys. Med. Biol.* **23,** 455–470.

Bateman, J. E., Connolly, J. F., Stephenson, R., Tappen, G. J. R. and Flesher, A. C. (1983). The development of MWPC-based systems for imaging X-rays, gamma rays and charged particles in applications in medicine, materials science and biochemistry. *Nucl. Instrum. Methods* **217,** 77–88.

Bender, M. A. and Blau, M. (1963). The autofluoroscope. *Nucleonics* **21,** 52–56.

Chang, L. T., Kaplan, S. N., Macdonald, B., Perez-Mendez, V. and Shiraishi, L. (1974). A method of tomographic imaging using a multiple pinhole coded aperture. *J. Nucl. Med.* **15,** 1063–1065.

Chu, D., Tam, K., Perez-Mendez, V., Kaplan, S. N., Lim, C., Hattner, R., Kaufman, L., Price, D. and Swann, S. (1977). High efficiency gamma converters and their application in an MWPC positron camera. *In* "Medical Radionuclide Imaging", Vol. 1, pp. 171–193. IAEA, Vienna.

Crawley, J. C. W., Ajdukiewicz, A. B., Bassett, N., Cronquist, A. G. and Veall, N. (1981). A radioisotope scanner for use in developing countries. *In* "Medical Radionuclide Imaging", Vol. 1, pp. 73–82. IAEA, Vienna.

Crippin, D. D. M. (1976). Single sideband methods in Fresnel zone plate imaging. *In* "Information Processing in Scintigraphy" (C. Raynaud and A. Todd-Pokropek, eds.), pp. 446–454. Service de Documentation du CEN Saclay, No. 76–003.

Davis, T. P. and Martonne, R. J. (1966). The hybrid radioisotope scanner. *J. Nucl. Med.* **7,** 114–128.

Detko, J. (1969). Semiconductor diode matrix for isotope localization. *Phys. Med. Biol.* **14,** 245–253.

Driard, B., Guyot, L. F. and Verat, M. (1971). A 35 cm input-field image intensifier for scintillation cameras. *Adv. Electron.*, **33,** 1031–1039.

Everett, D. B., Fleming, J. S., Todd. R. W. and Nightingale, J. M. (1976). A camera using Compton interactions. *In* "Medical Images: Formation, Perception and Measurement" (G. A. Hay, ed.), pp. 89–98. Institute of Physics and John Wiley, Bristol.

Jeavons, A. P., Charpak, G. and Stubbs, R. J. (1975). The high-density multiwire drift chamber. *Nucl. Instrum. Methods* **124,** 491–503.

Jeavons, A. P, Townsend, D. W., Ford N. I. and Kull, K. (1978). A high-resolution proportional chamber positron camera and its applications. *IEEE Trans. Nuc. Sci.* **NS-25,** 164–173.

Kaufman, L., Lorenz, V., Hosier, K., Hoenninger, J., Hattner, R. S., Okerlund, M., Price, D. C., Shames, D. M., Swann, S. J., Ewins, J. H., Armantrout, G. A., Camp, D. C. and Lee, K. (1978). Two-detector, 512-element high purity germanium camera prototype. *IEEE Trans. Nucl. Sci.* **NS-25,** 189–195.

Kellershohn, C. and Pellerin, P. (1955). Sur la possibilité d'utiliser un tube amplificateur d'image pour mettre en évidence la localisation et la distribution d'un corps radioactif. *C. R. Seances Soc. Biol. Ses Fil.* **149,** 533–536.

Keyes, W. I. (1975). The fan-beam gamma-camera. *Phys. Med. Biol.* **20,** 489–493.

Koral, K. F., Rogers, W. L. and Knoll, G. F. (1975). Digital tomographic imaging with time-modulated pseudorandom coded aperture and Anger camera. *J. Nucl. Med.* **16,** 402–413.

Macovski, A. (1974). Gamma ray imaging system using modulated apertures. *Phys. Med. Biol.* **19,** 523–533.

Mitchell, J. G., Mallard, J. R., Egerton, I. B., Caldwell, A. B., Lakshmanan, A. V., Nunan, C. and Turnbull, W. (1973). Towards a fine-resolution image-intensifier gamma-camera: the Abergammascope. *In* "Medical Radioisotope Scintigraphy", Vol. 1, pp. 157–167. IAEA, Vienna.

Mulder, H. and Pauwels, E. K. U. (1976). A new nuclear medicine scintillation camera based on image-intensifier tubes. *J. Nucl. Med.* **17,** 1008–1012.

Parker, R. P., Gunnersen, E. M., Ellis, R. and Bell, J. (1973). A semi-conductor gamma-camera: assessment of results. *In* "Medical Radioisotope Scintigraphy", Vol. 1, pp. 193–216. IAEA, Vienna.

Reading, D. H. (1976). Multiwire proportional chambers, *In* "Medical Images: Formation,

Perception and Measurement" (G. A. Hay, ed.), pp. 39–50. Institute of Physics and John Wiley, Bristol.

Roux, G., Gaucher, J. C., Lansiart, A. and Lequais, J. (1972). Detecteur photoelectronique analogique de la position de scintillations faiblement lumineuses. *In* "Photo-Electronic Image Devices", pp. 1017–1029, Academic Press, New York and London.

Singh, M. (1983). An electronically collimated gamma-camera for single photon emission computed tomography. Part 1: Theoretical considerations and design criteria. *Med. Phys.* **10,** 421–427.

Singh, M. and Doria, D. (1983). An electronically collimated gamma-camera for single photon emission tomography. Part II: Image reconstruction and preliminary experimental measurements. *Med. Phys.* **10,** 428–435.

Todd, P. W., Nightingale, J. M. and Everett, D. B. (1974). A proposed gamma-camera. *Nature (London)* **251,** 132–134.

Chapter 7

Image Display

7.1 Introduction

In nuclear medicine, data are presented primarily as images, although
analytical descriptions provide useful supplementary information particularly when large numbers of images are involved, as in dynamic studies.
The analytical treatment of data will be discussed in detail in the next
chapter.

Since data handling by computer interfaced systems is widely used,
digital as well as the conventional analogue displays are employed.
Attempts to compensate for the intrinsically poor quality of radionuclide
images by mathematical manipulation of the digitised data has led to a
wide variety of display formats. The existence of so many different
methods of data presentation is as much a result of the difficulty in
measuring their effectiveness as an indication of their value. Nevertheless,
quantification of image quality is important not only for assessing displays
per se, but also as the final measure of imaging device performance.

7.2 Display systems

7.2.1 Analogue displays

The most widely used analogue display is the cathode ray tube (CRT)
display of the gamma camera. The analogue X and Y coordinate signals
corresponding to the location of the scintillation are applied to the

deflection plates of the tube; if the energy (Z signal) of the event is accepted by the pulse height analyser, an unblank signal switches on the beam for a few microseconds. Each detected gamma ray thus appears as a flash of light on the tube face and a permanent image is produced by integrating these flashes on photographic film (see, for example, Fig. 2.11).

The main problem with this type of display is choosing the correct exposure for the film. Exposure will depend upon the brightness of the beam, the image count density as well as the type of recording film used.

Polaroid instant print film and single-side emulsion transparency film are the two main recording media. Polaroid is popular as it combines high speed (3000 ASA for black and white, Type 107C) with high resolution. As the finished print is available within 30 sec of exposure, then in the event of an incorrect exposure the study can be repeated before the patient has left the examination room. However, Polaroid film is expensive, has poor contrast (film gamma = 1.3) and has limited dynamic range. One solution to this latter problem has been to use a triple-lens camera to produce simultaneouly three images at different exposures, but this will only give very small images.

In many centres Polaroid film has been replaced by transparency film which can be developed in the standard X-ray rapid processor. While lacking the simplicity of Polaroid, it will provide an image within a few minutes of exposure. Conventional X-ray film has emulsion on both sides of a support film in order to record data from the intensifying screens at the front and back of the X-ray cassette, but such an arrangement is unnecessary when recording a CRT image and even counterproductive in that it may produce blurring. Special nuclear medicine film has emulsion only on one side of the support film, the rear being covered by an antihalation backing to reduce light scattering.

Transparency film is available in sizes up to 11×14 in^2 and while it is probably of little advantage to produce a single image of this size (see Section 7.2.2.3) these dimensions do allow several images to be recorded on the single sheet of film. Multi-formatting systems vary in sophistication from a manual type in which a slide is moved to allow only a small area of the film to be exposed at any one time, to those which can produce up to 81 images on a sheet, simultaneously record images at two different intensities and automatically record sequential images in a dynamic study.

7.2.2　Digital displays

When image data are to be handled by a computer-interfaced display system, the analogue coordinate signals must be digitised, with the result that the image appears as a regular array of picture elements or pixels.

Image intensity, the number of counts per pixel, is represented by either a range of grey shades or colours (Fig. 7.1a).

This digital display has many advantages over the analogue. In particular, since the image is non-volatile it can be manipulated prior to viewing by, for example, altering contrast and thresholding off unwanted background counts. It also permits quantitative information to be produced as well as sophisticated forms of image processing. These will be discussed in the next chapter.

The main disadvantage of this type of display is that the image may be degraded by the digitisation of spatial and intensity information.

7.2.2.1 Image pixellation

Most commercial systems allow images to be digitised into arrays of 256×256 pixels or even 512×512, although there may be restrictions on image manipulation above 128×128. Choice of pixel size affects both the amount of store occupied by an image and the maximum rate at which data can be collected in a dynamic study. While both can be optimised by using an array with a small number of pixels, image quality will suffer since there will be a coarse spatial sampling of the original analogue signal; for example, compare Fig. 7.1a and Fig. 7.1d. Sampling theory (Nyquist's theorem) states , that in order to record all the spatial detail in the image, the data should be sampled at twice the highest spatial frequency present (see, e.g., Pratt, 1978). For imaging systems, the MTF may be used to decide the highest spatial frequency which should be adequately sampled. Metz and colleagues (1972) have advocated this approach for radiographic images, the frequency limit being that at which the error in the MTF is no more than 0.5%. This means in practice that the limit is the frequency at which the experimentally determined MTF drops to 0.5%. Typically, this suggests that, for a modern gamma camera, a pixel of 3 mm side length should be adequate, which for a 40-cm field of view corresponds to a 128×128 array.

In radionuclide images one further physical factor must be considered, namely the degree of statistical noise. Reduction of pixel size in an effort to improve spatial detail causes the mean number of counts per pixel to decrease too, resulting in greater statistical noise. This may, therefore, lead to the use of a pixel size larger than that suggested by spatial sampling.

Apart from physical criteria, one must also consider the effect of pixel size on the visual appearance of the image. The coarser the pixellation the more obvious it is that the image is made up of a regular array of distinct elements (Fig. 7.1). It is the need to avoid this 'perceptual noise' that provides the impetus for using very fine pixellation, not the ability to extract a more faithful reproduction of the object.

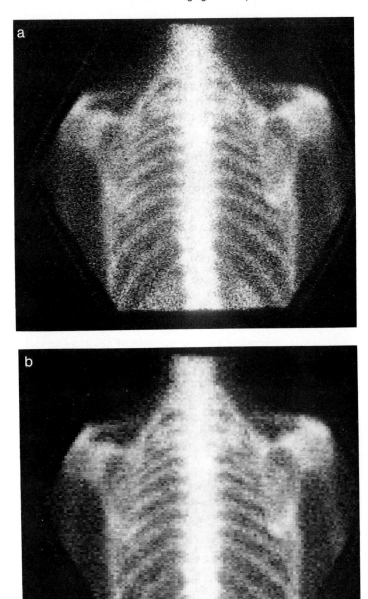

Fig. 7.1. Bone scan digitised into different numbers of picture elements. (a) 256 × 256, (b) 128 × 128, (c) 64 × 64 and (d) 32 × 32.

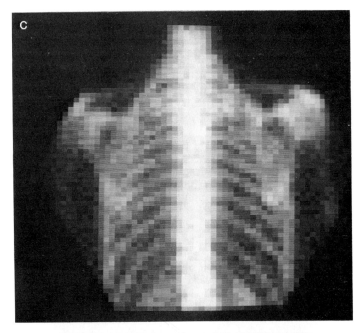

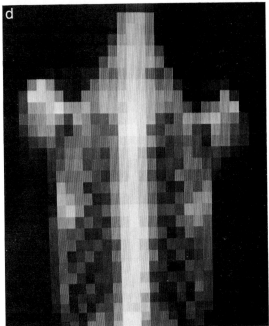

FIG. 7.1 (*Continued*)

Since the use of fine pixellation limits data acquisition and manipulation, it is worth considering how this may be avoided. There are two possibilities: data interpolation and image minification.

7.2.2.2 Interpolation

This involves using mathematical algorithms to predict the intensity values of pixels at points between those at which the data were acquired. Bilinear interpolation is the simplest and most widely used (Fig. 7.2a). The count density of the interpolated pixels is taken to be the arithmetic mean of the nearest-neighbour pixels. The sine function interpolation (Todd-Pokropek and Pizer, 1977) provides a mathematically more precise result, although it apparently makes little difference to image quality.

As can be seen by comparing Fig. 7.1b and Fig. 7.2a, the effect of interpolation is to introduce a degree of smoothing into the data as the value at the interpolated point is derived from those of the surrounding pixels. Sharp *et al.* (1982) suggest that this visual effect could be overcome by injecting appropriate random noise into the interpolated pixel values. The intensity value I for the interpolated pixel is first calculated by bilinear interpolation. This value is replaced by a random number generated in the range $I \pm k\sqrt{I}$ where k is a constant and $\sqrt{I}$ is the standard deviation of I, assuming that it is a Poisson variable. A value of $k = 1$ was found to be optimal (Fig. 7.2b).

While this procedure can in no way be said to be improving image fidelity, indeed image noise is increased, it may improve the visual acceptability of the image to the observer. Sharp *et al.* (1982) showed that, for simple test patterns, interpolation had no effect on an observer's ability to interpret the image, yet when faced with a selection of clinical images the observer preferred interpolated images to the original ones and random interpolation to bilinear. Indeed at fine pixellation, where noise was high, images interpolated to produce a small pixel were preferred to those acquired directly with the small pixel. Interpolation retains the mean count density of the original, coarser pixellation, and so count density is a factor of four higher than in the image acquired with the small pixel.

7.2.2.3 Minification

The human visual system does not respond equally well to all spatial frequencies but has a transfer function peaking at a few cycles per degree (Campbell, 1980). If it can be arranged that the frequencies of interest in the image coincide with the band of optimally perceived frequencies, then it should be possible to enhance the signal and at the same time reduce the interference from the higher frequencies of the pixel matrix.

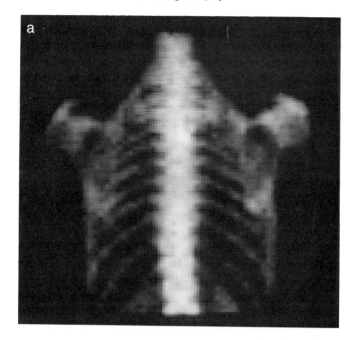

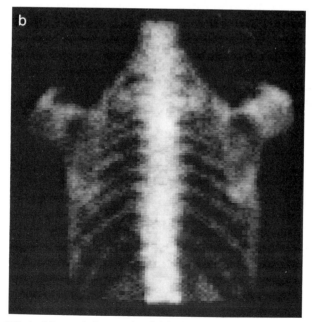

FIG. 7.2. Effect of interpolation on the digitised bone image of Fig. 7.1. (a) An image originally acquired on a 64×64 after simple bilinear interpolation into a 128×128 matrix. (b) Random interpolation into a 128×128 matrix.

The simplest way to vary the visual angle of the image is to alter the distance from which the image is viewed, an experiment the reader can try by looking at Fig. 7.1 from different distances. Pitt *et al.* (1983) demonstrated that observers could see no difference between the quality of bone images displayed on a 128×128 and 256×256 matrix at viewing distances between 4 and 12 m, the 128×128 matrix subtending a visual angle of 1.4 min of arc at 12 m. When the number of lesions which could be detected in an image was recorded, again a 128×128 matrix gave results as good as, or better than, a 256×256 matrix. However, the optimum viewing distance depended upon the size of the lesion: for an 8-cm-square image the best results were obtained by first viewing it from 1 m and then taking a pace backwards and viewing it from 2 m.

7.2.2.4 *Intensity coding*

The number of counts in a pixel can be displayed by coding it into either colour or grey shades. The most frequently employed method is linear mapping (Fig. 7.3a) whereby the range of counts per pixel in the image is divided into a number of equal-width bands, and those pixels with counts inside the same band are displayed at the same intensity level. The number

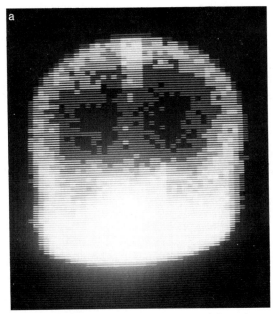

FIG. 7.3. Brain scan displayed with different types of intensity coding. (a) Linear mapping, (b) statistical banding and (c) histogram equalisation.

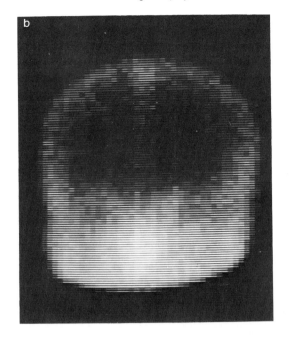

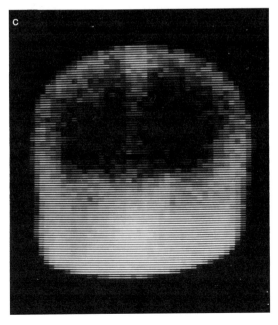

FIG. 7.3. (*Continued*)

of intensity levels available varies between systems, typically ranging from 16 to 256. At the high end of this range it may be possible to denote a change of only 1 count/pixel by a different intensity level, but such a display may not necessarily be optimal as statistical noise accounts for many count density changes. A smaller number of intensity levels may reduce displayed noise but it should be noted that if too large a range of count density is represented by an intensity level, significant changes may fail to appear as an intensity change in the displayed image and quality will suffer (Sharp and Mallard, 1976).

As has already been mentioned, the main advantage of a digital display system is that it allows the operator to vary rapidly the way in which data are displayed by changing contrast, thresholding, etc. Such an interactive procedure carried out conscientiously will probably ensure that maximum information is extracted. However, it is probably still prudent to ensure that the initial presentation of the image is close to optimum and several non-linear mapping schemes have been proposed to achieve this.

7.2.2.4.1   Statistical banding

If it is assumed that the main contribution to image noise is statistical fluctuation in the count density, then perceived noise can be controlled by choosing the width of each intensity level so that only statistically significant changes in count density cause a change in display intensity. In practice, as the mean count density of the image varies from area to area, it is not possible to implement a genuine statistical coding system, and instead one is used in which the width of a band is chosen to be a constant number of standard deviations of the mean count density associated with that band. Figure 7.3b shows an image coded with two standard deviation wide statistical bands.

Sharp and Mallard (1976) showed that for a simple test pattern the width of a band should not exceed three standard deviations. It is, of course, possible to express the widths of bands in a linear coding system in units of standard deviations of the mean count density of that band, although, in contrast to the statistical system, the number of standard deviations within the band will vary from band to band, being smallest at the high count density end of the scale. However, if information is not to be lost the linear scale must not have a bandwidth greater than three standard deviations at any point.

7.2.2.4.2   Histogram equalisation

In a linear banding system the distribution of intensity levels reflects the range of count density in the image with the result that most levels will be associated with areas of high count density, leaving few for coding the rest of the image. This creates a difficulty in brain images, for example (Fig.

7.3a), where there is a high count density over facial muscles, salivary glands, etc., whilst the more important brain tissue contains little activity. In the histogram equalisation algorithm (Goris *et al.*, 1976), levels are chosen such that each display intensity appears the same number of times in the image (Fig. 7.3c). Of course this also has the possible disadvantage that if too few intensity levels are used then isolated areas of high count density may not be adequately displayed.

7.2.2.4.3 Minimisation of uncertainty

Cormack and Hutton (1980) suggested that an optimum coding system could be produced by considering the display process as a series of information channels. The transfer of information from one stage in the process to another could then be measured in terms of information transfer I, which denotes the resulting change in uncertainty or entropy H (see, e.g., Brillouin, 1956). In particular, display coding is concerned with the uncertainty $H_{ij}(\Lambda/\rho)$ about the true value (mean) λ of the number of counts in pixel (i,j) given that it is seen by the observer as being displayed with an intensity level ρ.

An optimum coding system, they suggested, would be one which minimised the mean pixel uncertainty H_{mean} in the image

$$H_{\text{mean}} = \frac{1}{N}\sum_{ij} H_{ij}(\Lambda|\rho) \qquad \text{bits per pixel} \qquad (7.1)$$

N being the total number of pixels in the image. According to information theory, uncertainty is given by

$$H(\Lambda|\rho) = -\int_0^\infty p(\lambda|\rho)\log_2[p(\lambda|\rho)]d\lambda \qquad \text{bits} \qquad (7.2)$$

being the set of all possible values λ for the true number of counts in a pixel.

From Bayes' theorem

$$p(\lambda|\rho) = p(\rho|\lambda)p(\lambda) \Big/ \int_0^\infty p(\rho|\lambda)p(\lambda)\,d\lambda \qquad (7.3)$$

$p(\lambda)$ being the *a priori* probability that the true pixel value is λ. In the general case where there is no prior knowledge about the distribution of counts in the image then it is equally probable that λ will take any positive value.

The term $p(\rho/\lambda)$, the probability that a mean count of λ will produce an intensity level ρ, depends on the upper and lower count density limits of the ρth intensity level, U_ρ and L_ρ, and the probability $p(n/\lambda)$ that there will be n counts in the pixel. This latter probability is given by the Poisson statistic

$$p(n|\lambda) = e^{-\lambda}\lambda^n/n! \tag{7.4}$$

hence

$$p(\rho|\lambda) = \sum_{n=L_\rho}^{U_\rho} \frac{e^{-\lambda}\lambda^n}{n!} \tag{7.5}$$

substituting Eq. (7.5) in Eq. (7.2) gives

$$H(\Lambda|\rho) = \log_2(U_\rho - L_\rho) - \frac{1}{U_\rho - L_\rho} \int_0^\infty \left(\sum_{n=L_\rho}^{U_\rho} \frac{e^{-\lambda}\lambda^n}{n!} \right)$$

$$\times \log_2 \left(\sum_{n=L_\rho}^{U_\rho} \frac{e^{-\lambda}\lambda^n}{n!} \right) d\lambda \tag{7.6}$$

This allows H_{mean} to be minimised by varying U_ρ and L_ρ.

It has been assumed that the perceived intensity level P is the same as that in which the data is coded, say k, i.e.,

$$p(\rho|k) = \delta(\rho - k)$$

The measurement of this relationship between perceived and displayed intensity provides a way of assessing display performance. In the case where an equivalence cannot be assumed, Eq. (7.6) becomes (Cormack and Hutton, 1981)

$$H(\Lambda|\rho) = \log_2 \sum_{k=1}^{M} p(\rho|k)[U_K - L_K]$$

$$- \int_0^\infty \left[\sum_{k=1}^{M} p(\rho|k)p(k|\lambda) \right] \log_2[p(\rho|k)p(k|\lambda)]d\lambda \Big/ \sum_{k=1}^{M} p(\rho|k)[U_k - L_k]$$

$$\tag{7.7}$$

where M is the number of display levels.

An example of an image displayed with this coding is shown in Fig. 7.4. In many circumstances the coding is similar to that produced by histogram equalisation.

7.2.2.4.4 Representation of intensity

Intensity can be represented either by colour or grey shades, the latter being the most popular as they give a coding sequence which is easily understood. Unfortunately, there are only a limited number of grey levels which are readily perceptible as being different, although varying display contrast may increase this number. On the other hand, colour scales can be

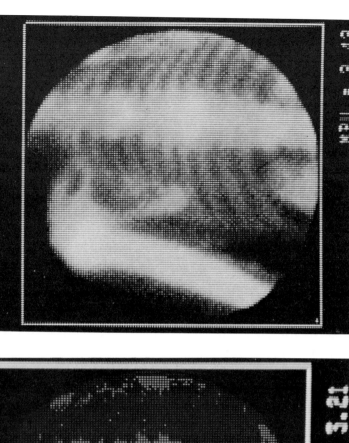

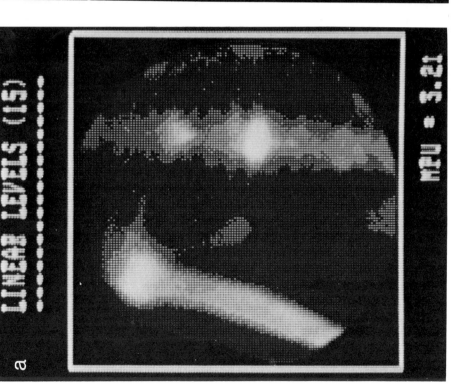

Fig. 7.4. Posterior bone image. (a) Intensity coded into 15 linear levels. (b) Intensity coded into 15 levels using minimisation of mean pixel uncertainty. (Courtesy of Mr. B. Hulton.)

chosen so that highly contrasting colours are used for adjacent levels, and, hence, a large number of levels can be used. Unfortunately this has the disadvantage of depriving the visual system of the power of associability (Cormack and Hutton, 1980), i.e., seeing adjacent intensity levels as possibly relating to the same image feature. Instead the observer is very aware of the contours formed by pixels coded with the same colour.

To utilise the extended dynamic range offered by colour coding whilst avoiding, to a large extent, the problem of associability, colour scales have been proposed in which differences in saturation are used to denote intensity changes rather than changes in hue. The heated body spectrum (Milan and Taylor, 1975) (Fig. 7.5) is an example of this scale, the colour code varying from black through shades of red, orange, yellow and ending in white.

In the geographical coding scale (Houston, 1980), four distinct hues are used (blue, green, yellow and red) with intermediate intensity levels produced by varying the degree of saturation of each colour (Fig. 7.5). Whilst for any one colour this acts as a pseudoanalogue coding, the contours produced by the abrupt change from, say, the most saturated blue level to the least saturated green are highly distracting. In a comparison of intensity scales, using a linear coding system, Houston (1980) found the heated body spectrum to be best, closely followed by the grey shade, with

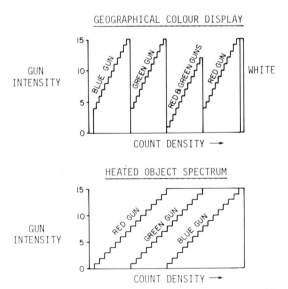

Fig. 7.5. Colour coding systems. The displayed colour is determined by the intensity of each of the three colour guns on the TV display. [From Houston (1980).]

the geographical scale worst. The contrasting colour scale was not included.

One situation in which the contrasting colour scale has a definite advantage is in coding the image to show absolute, rather than relative, quantitative information as in functional imaging, for example.

While the advantage of digital displays lies in providing interactive data presentation, hard-copy images are frequently required for insertion in a patient's notes and for presentation at ward conferences. Multiformatting devices are probably the best way to copy a grey scale image, although directly photographing the television screen is acceptable. The cheapest way to produce a colour image is with an electromechanical colour printer, but such systems are slow in operation, the choice of colours is limited and the final hard copy is frequently of disappointing quality. Ink jet printers are a possible alternative but have not yet been proved reliable. Electrostatic printers are adequate for reproducing graphical information such as time–activity curves from dynamic studies but are not satisfactory for image reproduction.

7.3 Image evaluation

The problem of assessing display performance as part of a quality control procedure has already been discussed in Chapter 5. The more general problem of judging the quality of the image goes beyond simply ensuring display fidelity.

Measures of image quality can be either objective or subjective. The latter involves perceptual measurements taken with an observer viewing a test pattern. The former does not, but may use a mathematical model of the perceptual process.

7.3.1 Objective measures

For imaging systems in which noise can be neglected, quality indices have concentrated upon image sharpness.

Linfoot (1964) defined the fidelity of an image in terms of the squared difference between the intensities of image $i(x,y)$ and object $o(x,y)$.

$$\text{Image fidelity} = 1 - \left\{ \int\!\!\int [o(x,y) - i(x,y)]^2 \, dx \, dy \Big/ \int\!\!\int o(x,y)^2 \, dx \, dy \right\}$$

$$(7.8)$$

For a good image, fidelity would tend to unity. Linfoot also proposed that quality could be measured by the correlation between object and image

$$\text{Correlation quality} = \int\int o(x,y)i(x,y)\,dx\,dy \left/ \int\int o(x,y)^2\,dx\,dy \right. \qquad (7.9)$$

A third measure suggested was relative structural content, a measure of the capacity to reproduce fine detail

$$\text{Relative structural content} = \int\int i(x,y)^2\,dx\,dy \left/ \int\int o(x,y)^2\,dx\,dy \right. \quad (7.10)$$

In fact these measures are not independent:

Image fidelity + relative structural content = 2 × correlation quality

If it can be assumed that the object has the structure of white Gaussian noise, then (Wagner and Weaver, 1973)

$$\text{Relative structural content} = \int\int \text{MTF}(f_x, f_y)^2 df_x\, df_y \qquad (7.11)$$

where MTF is the system's modulation transfer function. This measure is equivalent to what Schade (1956) has called the noise equivalent passband (NEP). This index, it is claimed, correlates well with the subjective impression of image sharpness.

The mean square gradient of the density distribution across the image of a sharp edge, the acutance, is also found to correlate with sharpness. Acutance is defined as

$$\frac{1}{\Delta D}\left[\frac{1}{\Delta x}\int\left(\frac{dD}{dx}\right)^2 dx\right] \qquad (7.12)$$

and is approximately equal to $(2\Delta D/\Delta x)$ NEP at low contrasts, where ΔD and Δx are the range of density and the distance across the edge, respectively.

In most clinical radionuclide images, noise must be considered to have an effect at least as great as that of sharpness on quality and any useful measure of quality must take noise into account. Two types of noise are present; the statistical (Poisson) fluctuations in count density and 'anatomical' noise resulting from uncertainty as to the normal distribution pattern of the radiopharmaceutical.

In the search for objective measures of image quality it is of value to consider models of the process by which detail may be perceived in noisy images.

7.3.1.1 *Models of visual detection*

The visual analysis of an image can be considered to take place at three levels:

   (i)   detection: the realisation that there is an abnormality in the image

   (ii)   recognition: the process of being able to describe the abnormality in terms of size, shape, etc.

   (iii)   identification: a complete classification of the abnormality.

Most models of the perceptual process have been limited to detection, in particular the ability to detect an isolated detail (the signal) amongst a background of statistical noise.

De Vries (1943) and Rose (1946) were the first to suggest that the ratio of signal to noise (SNR) was the major factor in determining the quality of photon-limited images. They proposed a model in which the background noise was sampled over some area A equal in size to the signal. If the image has a mean of N photons per unit area and the signal $(N + \Delta N)$ per unit area, then for the signal to be detected

$$\Delta NA = k \sqrt{NA} \qquad (7.13)$$

where $\sqrt{NA}$ is the noise in the background, assuming that it is Poisson distributed, and k is a constant, the SNR. For the signal to be detected then its minimum contrast C is given by

$$C = \Delta N/N = k/\sqrt{NA} \qquad (7.14)$$

Rose suggested that k had a value of between 3 and 5.

The ideas inherent in this model have been extended by later workers. For example, Morgan (1965) suggested that the sample area A should be determined by the transfer function of the visual system rather than signal size

$$A = \left[\int \int \mathrm{MTF}(f_x, f_y)^2 \, df_x \, df_y \right]^{-1} \qquad (7.15)$$

Thus Morgan's sample area is equal to the inverse of the noise equivalent passband.

Schade (1956) presented a more general approach in which each element i in the imaging system contributed its own effective sampling area $\bar{a}_i$, defined as in Eq. (7.15). The total sampling area is then calculated simply from the sum of the individual areas. While more sophisticated models based on the statistical test have been devised, it is worth considering the philosophy of this model.

The statistical approach adopted by theories like that of Rose is that once the signal intensity exceeds some limiting value determined by the average behaviour of the noise, then the signal will be seen. In practice, perception of the signal will depend upon whether the noise in a particular image fluctuates sufficiently to produce at least one area which may be confused with the signal. Thus, at a particular contrast the signal may be seen in one image but not in another, and so signal detectability can only be expressed as a probability.

If we consider our problem of detecting an area of increased count density in a background of constant mean count density, then the probability of correctly detecting the signal is given by (Sharp and Mallard, 1974).

$$\sum_i (\text{Probability that the signal has an intensity } i)$$

$$\times \begin{array}{l} [\text{Probability that the background contains} \\ \text{no area of intensity exceeding } (i - d)] \end{array} \qquad (7.16)$$

The problem is now reduced to one of comparing the signal with likely alternatives in the background. It is still necessary to postulate that some minimum intensity difference d must occur for one possibility to be regarded as more likely than another. The value for d would depend upon type of display used and the confidence with which an observer gives a positive response (see Section 7.3.2.2).

Decision theory offers another approach to modelling perceptual performance. Given a set of readings $(x_1, x_2, x_3, \ldots)$, which in this case would constitute the image, the likelihood L that these originate from the probability distribution $f_s(x)$, describing the signal is defined as

$$L(S) = \prod_i f_s(x_i) \qquad (7.17)$$

Similarly, the likelihood that the readings originated from the noise distribution $f_N(x)$ is

$$L(N) = \prod_i f_N(x_i) \qquad (7.18)$$

If it is equally probable that the readings were signal or were noise then a decision should be made in favour of the one having the larger likelihood. If we define the likelihood ratio as

$$LR = L(S)/L(N) \qquad (7.19)$$

then if $LR > 1$ the decision should be that the readings are from the signal.

It can be shown (Peterson et al., 1954) that many decision strategies— e.g., maximising the percentage of correct decisions while keeping the

percentage of false positives below some predetermined level—
are equivalent to basing the decision on the value of the likelihood
ratio.

Swets *et al.* (1961) have suggested that the human observer makes
perceptual decisions using the likelihood ratio. The value that the ratio
must take if the observer is to 'see' the signal depends upon such factors as
a priori knowledge of the probability that a signal is present. Signal
detection theory will be discussed further in Section 7.3.2.2.

So far analysis of the image has been described in terms of the
magnitude of the signal and noise, and spatial structure has not been
considered. Structure is most easily introduced into the equations for the
SNR in terms of the amplitude spectrum of the Fourier transform of the
signal $S(f_x, f_y)$. Noise can be described by the Wiener spectrum WS (f_x, f_y)
or noise power spectrum. This is the Fourier transform of the auto-
correlation function of the background. The measurement and application
of the Wiener spectrum description of noise in radionuclide imaging is
described by Tsui *et al.* (1981).

The SNR for the likelihood ratio based detection process is given by

$$\mathrm{SNR}_L^2 = \int\int \frac{S(f_x, f_y)S^*(f_x, f_y)\, df_x\, df_y}{\mathrm{WS}(f_x, f_y)} \qquad (7.20)$$

where $S^*(f_x, f_y)$ is the complex conjugate.

Thus, it is only those noise frequencies within the frequency band of the
signal which mask it, i.e., it is noise resembling the signal which makes
detection difficult.

If the noise has no inherent spatial structure and is Gaussian, as, for
example, the statistical noise in a uniform background of radioactivity, the
Wiener spectrum has a constant value WS_0, the area under this curve being
equal to the noise variance.

In this case

$$\mathrm{SNR}_L^2 = \int S(f_x, f_y)S^*(f_x, f_y)\, df_x\, df_y \Big/ \mathrm{WS}_0 \qquad (7.21)$$

which is often abbreviated to

$$\mathrm{SNR}_L = \sqrt{E/\mathrm{WS}_0} \qquad (7.22)$$

where E is the energy or quadratic content of the signal.

In the case of the signal having a flat top, Eq. (7.21) is equivalent to that
obtained from Rose's theory.

7.3.2   Subjective measurement

The measurement of an observer's ability to detect a signal (the abnormality) in the presence of noise is a classical problem in psychophysics and several experimental techniques have been developed. Of particular relevance are the method of constant stimulus (Corso, 1967) and signal detection theory (Green and Swets, 1966).

7.3.2.1   The method of constant stimulus

This technique is best demonstrated by an example (Sharp and Mallard, 1976). It is clear from Section 2.1.1 that the effect of statistical noise on image quality can be reduced by increasing the count density in the image. The problem we will consider is how to quantify the resulting improvement in quality.

A simple test pattern is used (Fig. 7.6) consisting of a uniform background of radioactivity with a single circular area of increased activity representing an abnormality. Image quality can then be measured by the observer's ability to discriminate between the abnormality and statistical noise.

With the method of constant stimulus, the observer is presented with a set of images for each selected value of the background count density. In each set, the contrast of the abnormality, in this case defined as the ratio of the peak count density in the abnormality to the mean background count density, is varied from a maximum value at which it is clearly detectable, to some minimum value at which it cannot be distinguished from noise. At each contrast value several repeat images are taken, the location of the abnormality being varied. Since the noise is random, repeated images can show marked variations in appearance (Fig. 7.6). The percentage of images in which an observer can correctly detect the abnormality is known as the observer's true positive visual response. A plot of this visual response against image contrast gives the visual response curve. If the range of contrast has been correctly chosen, visual response will vary between 100%, the abnormality at this contrast being always detected, and 0%.

The method is shown diagrammatically in Fig. 7.7. The variability in visual impression produced by images of the same contrast is denoted by probability curves, curves 1–3 being associated with three different levels of contrast. It is assumed that the observer adopts some visual threshold T such that if the visual impression produced by an image exceeds T the observer reports that an abnormality is present. The proportion of the area under a probability curve which falls to the right of T equals the observer's

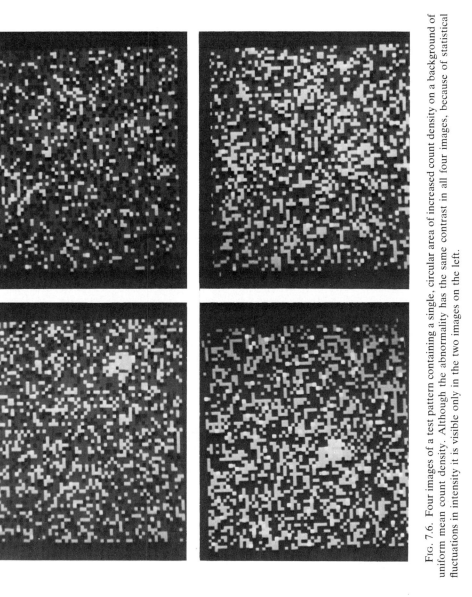

Fig. 7.6. Four images of a test pattern containing a single, circular area of increased count density on a background of uniform mean count density. Although the abnormality has the same contrast in all four images, because of statistical fluctuations in intensity it is visible only in the two images on the left.

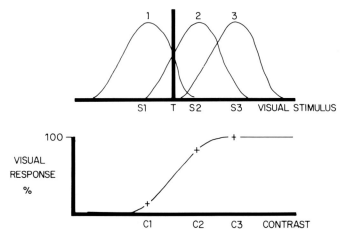

FIG. 7.7. Principle of the method of constant stimulus.

true positive visual response to a set of images of this contrast. As contrast increases, the images produce a greater impression of containing an abnormality and so the curves fall further to the right of T and give a higher true positive visual response.

Figure 7.8 shows the visual response curves produced by six observers. There is some observer variation in defining a perceptible abnormality so the curves are not identical. In order to express image quality by a single number, the average contrast which elicits a 50% visual response was chosen. This value has been called the detection contrast; note from Fig. 7.7 that this value corresponds to the visual threshold T. Figure 7.9 shows how detection contrast decreased, i.e., image quality improved, as the background count density increased. For this particular display, detection contrast was inversely proportional to the square root of the background count density.

7.3.2.2 Signal detection theory

One of the main problems in a perceptual experiment is defining an observer's decision criterion, i.e., how certain the observer should be before classifying an image as abnormal. Differences in their understanding of what constitutes an abnormal image cause observers to adopt different visual thresholds, and so their visual response curves differ (Fig. 7.8). When using the method of constant stimulus, this raises the possibility that changes in detection contrast may be produced by variations in the decision criterion used by an observer rather than by real changes in image quality. Signal detection theory attempts to overcome

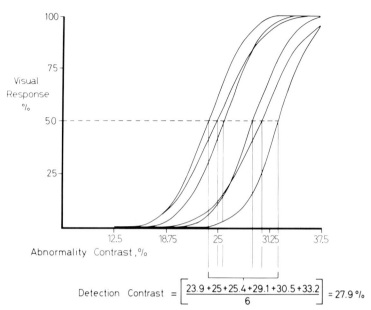

FIG. 7.8. Visual response curves from six observers who have been presented with the same set of images. Detection contrast has been calculated as the average contrast producing a 50% visual response.

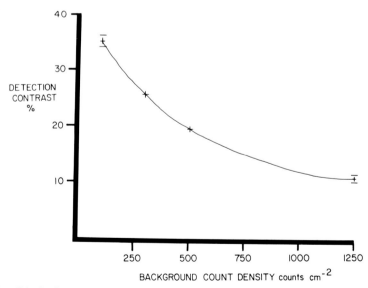

FIG. 7.9. Performance of a digital display using statistical grey level intensity coding, expressed in terms of how the detection contrast changed with the background count density.

this problem as shown in Fig. 7.10. If the observer gives a positive response even when he has only a slight suspicion that the image may contain an abnormality, he is using a low visual threshold such as A (Fig. 7.10). Since the probability curve representing abnormal images S falls mainly to the right of A, there will be a high true positive visual response rate from the observer. On the other hand, if he is very cautious and only reports as abnormal those images which are obviously abnormal, then he is using a high visual threshold E, and the corresponding true positive visual response rate will be low. If the observer is presented with normal images (curve N), as well as abnormal ones, there is a high probability that when using threshold A he will call some normal images abnormal, i.e., he mistakenly identifies noise as an abnormality. This is known as a false positive response. When the observer is being cautious (threshold E), the probability of a false positive response is very low.

The first problem is how to persuade an observer to change his visual threshold, the resulting variation of true positive response rate (area of curve S to the right of the threshold) with false positive response rate (area of curve N to the right of the threshold) will show to what extent the two probability curves overlap. This overlap indicates how well the abnormal images can be distinguished from the normal ones, i.e., it measures the quality of the image produced by the display.

The first problem is how to persuade an observer to use different visual thresholds. One commonly-employed method is to ask the observer to assign a confidence rating to each of his positive responses (Green and

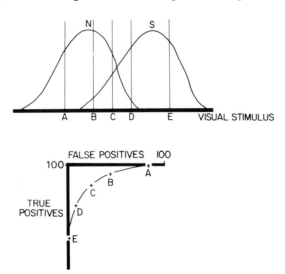

FIG. 7.10. Principle of signal detection theory.

Swets, 1966), using some predefined scale such as that shown in Table 7.1. If the observer is absolutely certain that the image is abnormal, he gives it a rating of 5, while if he thinks that what he sees is almost certainly noise then he rates his response as 1. Ratings 1 to 5 can be thought to correspond to threshold E to A, respectively; thus using a rating is equivalent to employing five different visual thresholds simultaneously.

The curve showing how the true positive response varies with false positive response is known as the receiver operating characteristic (ROC) curve. Note that the points on the curve are not simply the percentage of true and false positive responses corresponding to a particular rating, since an image given a rating of 4, for example, not only exceeds threshold B but also C, D and E. Thus

$$TP_B = TP(1) + TP(2) + TP(3) + TP(4)$$

$$FP_B = FP(1) + FP(2) + FP(3) + FP(4)$$

where TP_B and FP_B are the true and false positive responses when threshold B is used and $TP(i)$ and $FP(i)$ are the responses corresponding to a rating i.

When it is not possible to distinguish between normal and abnormal images, i.e., when curves N and S are identical, the ROC curve becomes a straight line running from the bottom left-hand corner to the top-right hand one (Fig. 7.11). All responses are purely guessing. As it becomes easier to discriminate between the two groups, then the ROC curve shifts towards the upper left-hand corner of the graph.

If it can be assumed that the probability curves S and N are Gaussian with the same standard deviation, then the ROC curve is fully described by a single index, usually called d', which is the ratio of the separation of the mean of S and of N to their standard deviation; d' is thus a signal to noise ratio. Also in this particular case the slope of the ROC curve at any point is equal to the value of the likelihood ratio used to make the decision resulting in that combination of true and false positive responses.

TABLE 7.1. Description of the confidence ratings used to produce an ROC curve.

Rating	Description
5	Abnormality definitely present
4	Abnormality almost certainly present
3	Abnormality possibly present
2	Abnormality probably not present
1	Abnormality almost certainly not present

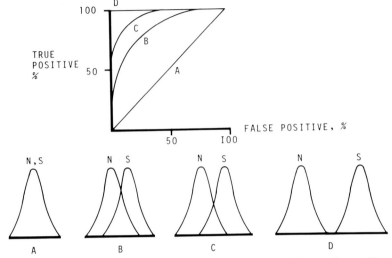

FIG. 7.11. How the separation between the normal and abnormal images (curves N and S, respectively) is reflected in the position of the ROC curve.

In these circumstances d' provides an ideal measure of device performance, specifying the discriminability between signal and noise alone since any changes in an observer's visual threshold (decision criterion) alters only the point at which his results will fall on the ROC curve and not the curve itself. Thus the differences between observers noted in Fig. 7.8 should not affect the value of d'.

However, the curves S and N are the signal and noise as perceived by the observer and so may be dependent upon his experience. Not all inter-observer differences are eradicated in practice, and indeed it has been suggested that signal detection theory provides a way of judging the effectiveness of training in image interpretation (Nishiyama *et al.*, 1975).

As far as perceptual measurements are concerned, it cannot be assumed that the probability distributions S and N have equal standard deviations and so d' cannot be used. Instead the area under the ROC curve is frequently adopted but unlike d' it does not provide a unique description of the curve.

The problem of measuring statistically the difference between two ROC curves is not simple, but solutions have been suggested (Dorfman and Alf, 1969; Metz and Kronman, 1980).

Simple signal detection theory is formulated to deal with only two classes of response, the image is normal or abnormal. In clinical radionuclide imaging, as in many other types of imaging, a correct response may also depend upon giving the true location for the abnormality. In this case there are three classes of response;

(i)   the true positive, correct location response which indicates that both the presence and location of the abnormality have been reported correctly

(ii)   the true positive, incorrect location response (an abnormality is present but not at the reported location)

(iii)   the false positive response, a positive response to an image which is normal.

The generalised ROC curve now has three axes (Fig. 7.12). The plot of the true positive, correct location responses against false positives is known as the localisation ROC, or LROC curve. Starr and colleagues (1975) have shown how the LROC curve may be calculated from the conventional ROC curve when the number of possible locations for the abnormality is known.

Simple signal detection theory is also concerned with the detection of a single abnormality while in many instances we are interested in images containing several possible abnormalities. Metz and colleagues (1976) showed that once again the shape of the curve obtained under these conditions could be predicted from the standard ROC curve.

A final problem facing the application of signal detection theory is when the number of lesions present varies from image to image but the observer has no knowledge of the number expected. If the observer is free to report any number of lesions in an image, it is not possible to calculate a false

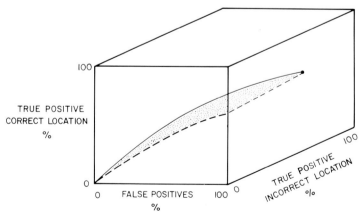

FIG. 7.12. Generalised ROC curve shown by the solid line. The LROC curve, the projection of the generalised curve onto the plane defined by the true positive correct location responses and the false positive responses, is shown by the dashed curve.

positive response rate since the maximum number of possible responses is not known. One suggested way of analysing such data is with the so-called free response ROC curve (Bunch *et al.*, 1977).

Unlike the method of constant stimulus, signal detection theory in its most general form only measures the ability to discriminate between two sets of data. In medical applications this is often sufficient since one set represents healthy and the other diseased patients. While signal detection theory reduces the psychological variability in an experiment, i.e., changes in visual threshold, it does so at the cost of providing information about the effect on image quality of varying the intensity of the abnormality. Of course, in situations where abnormality intensity cannot be readily defined and controlled by the experimentalist, signal detection theory is the only method that can be used. The methods of constant stimulus and signal detection theory are thus, in several respects, complementary techniques.

7.3.2.3 *Ranking/rating methods*

Both the method of constant stimulus and signal detection theory involve perceptual tasks requiring a specific binary response from the observer, the abnormality is either seen or not seen. While tasks can often be reduced to this form, nevertheless it does place a severe restriction on the range of problems which can be investigated.

It is often very easy for an experienced observer to say whether one image is better than another, yet difficult for him to define the criteria on which the judgement is based. Ranking techniques use this intuitive appreciation to measure the relative quality of a group of images. Each observer is given a set of images and asked to arrange them in order of preference: the image judged to be of highest quality to be ranked in first place, the next best second and so on. By comparing the ordering produced by several observers, it is possible to measure statistically whether they agree that images presented in one way are better than those shown in another way. This approach has, for example, been used in nuclear medicine to measure how pixel size affects the quality of digitised images (Sharp *et al.*, 1982).

The set of images used consisted of normal and abnormal bone, brain and liver scans, each image having been displayed with various pixellations. Each observer was shown a different set of these images. He was not told whether an image was normal or abnormal, nor was he asked to identify abnormalities but simply to rank the different pixellated versions of each image in order of preference. The number of occasions on which images presented with one particular pixellation were given a higher ranking than those of a different pixellation was noted. On the null hypothesis this number should be drawn from a binomial distribution in which there is equal probability of the ranking being higher or lower. Thus, it is possible to test whether there is a statistically significant difference in ranking order. The results of this experiment have been discussed in Section 7.2.2.2.

The main criticism of this approach is that the term 'preference' is imprecise. The technique is relying on the experience and even the prejudice of observers, in defining what constitutes a good image. However, the technique is very flexible with little restriction on the type of problem that can be investigated.

Of course, it is possible to define much more precisely the judgment criterion. For example, Kasal *et al.* (1983) used this technique to measure the smallest change in gamma-camera resolution which was perceptible in an image. The test pattern consisted of a high contrast straight edge which was imaged at different spatial resolutions. By comparing the number of occasions on which an image taken at one resolution was judged sharper than another, it was possible to decide when the change in resolution had produced a perceptible change in image quality.

Ranking can also be used to examine the correlation or agreement between objective measures of quality and subjective judgment. The images are first ranked by an observer and the ordering compared with that obtained by using the objective quality index, the degree of agreement being measured by Spearman's rank correlation coefficient.

Sharp and Marshall (1981) have used this method to look at the effectiveness of various measures of gamma-camera uniformity. Whilst one can measure whether there is good correlation between subjective and objective rankings, there is, unfortunately, no way of testing whether one correlation is better than another.

7.4 Concluding remarks

Whilst much effort has been expended on the design of gamma-cameras and on measuring their performance, relatively little attention has been given to the display. The basic principle of the display has changed very little from that used in Anger's original camera. Yet the performance of an imaging device is judged finally by the displayed image.

Digital technology has now developed sufficiently for it to be feasible, in economic as well as technical terms, to replace the analogue display with a digital one. The demands on such a display are not great, particularly as it appears that very fine digitisation of the image is unnecessary. There is the danger, however, that too much reliance will be placed upon interactive manipulation to give the best image. In a busy department this is unlikely to be carried out thoroughly and thought should be given to the design of software to produce a near optimal coding of the image intensity.

Undoubtedly the neglect of the display is due largely to the difficulty of measuring the effectiveness of image presentation. A simple mathematical measure of image quality, sufficiently general to be applied to radionuclide images, has yet to be produced. Experimental measurement of quality is often lengthy to perform, involving the viewing of many images, and this has probably deterred experimenters. The methodology for such subjective measurements is available and it is to be hoped that more work will be carried out in this field in the near future.

References

Brillouin, L. (1956). "Science and Information Theory". Academic Press, New York.

Bunch, P. C., Hamilton, J. F., Sanderson, G. K. and Simmons, H. F. (1977). A free response approach to the measurement and characterization of radiographic observer performance. *Proc. Soc. Photo-Opt. Instrum. Eng.* **127,** 124–135.

Campbell, F. W. (1980). The physics of visual perception. *Philos. Trans. R. Soc. London* **290,** 5–9.

Cormack, J. and Hutton, B. (1980). Minimisation of data transfer losses in the display of digitised scintigraphic images. *Phys. Med. Biol.* **25,** 271–282.

Cormack, J. and Hutton, B. F. (1981). Quantitation and optimization of digitised scintigraphic display characteristics using information theory. *In* "Medical Image Processing" (M. L. Goris, ed.), pp. 240–263. Stanford University Press, Stanford California.

Corso, J. F. (1967). "The Experimental Psychology of Sensory Behaviour", pp. 229–236. Holt, Rinehart & Winston, New York.

De Vries, H. L. (1943). The quantum character of light and its bearing upon threshold of vision, the differential sensitivity and visual acuity of the eye. *Physica (Amsterdam)* **10,** 553–564.

Dorfman, D. D. and Alf, E. (1969). Maximum likelihood estimation of parameters of signal-detection theory and determination of confidence intervals—ranking method data. *J. Math. Psychol.* **6,** 487–496.

Goris, M. L., Schiebe, P. O. and Kriss, J. R. (1976). A method to optimise the use of a greyshade scale in nuclear medicine images. *Comput. Biomed. Res.* **9,** 571–577.

Green, D. M. and Swets, J. A. (1966). "Signal Detection Theory and Psychophysics". John Wiley, New York.

Houston, A. S. (1980). A comparison of four standard scintigraphic TV displays. *J. Nucl. Med.* **21,** 512–517.

Kasal, B., Sharp, P. F. and Dendy, P. P. (1983). The relationship between objective and subjective assessment of gamma-camera image sharpness. *Phys. Med. Biol.* **28,** 1127–1134.

Linfoot, E. H. (1964). "Fourier Methods in Optical Image Evaluation", pp. 30–88. The Focal Press, London.

Metz, C. E. and Kronman, H. B. (1980). Statistical significance tests for binormal ROC curves. *J. Math. Psychol.* **22,** 218–243.

Metz, C. E., Strubler, K. A. and Rossman, K. (1972). Choice of line spread function sampling distance for computing the MTF of radiographic screen-film systems. *Phys. Med. Biol.* **17,** 638–647.

Metz, C. E., Starr, S. J. and Lusted, L. B. (1976). Observer performance in detecting multiple radiographic signals: prediction and analysis using a generalised ROC approach. *Radiology* **121,** 337–347.

Milan, J. and Taylor, K. J. W. (1975). The application of the temperature scale to ultrasound imaging. *J. Clin. Ultrasound* **3,** 171.

Morgan, R. H. (1965). Threshold visual perception and its relationship to photon fluctuations and sine-wave response. *Am. J. Roentgenol., Radium Ther. Nucl. Med.* **93,** 982–997.

Nishiyama, H., Lewis, J. T., Ashare, A. B. and Saenger, E. L. (1975). Interpretation of radionuclide liver images: Do training and experience make a difference? *J. Nucl. Med.* **16,** 11–16.

Peterson, W. W., Birdsall, T. G. and Fox, W. C. (1954). The theory of signal detectability. *Trans. IRE Prof. Group Inf. Theory* **PGIT-4,** 171–212.

Pitt, R. W., Sharp, P. F., Chesser, R. B. and Dendy, P. P. (1983). Radionuclide image minification can compensate for coarse digitization. *J. Nucl. Med.* **24,** 1046–1054.

Pratt, W. K. (1978). "Digital Image Processing", p. 97. John Wiley, Interscience, New York.

Rose, A. (1946). A unified approach to the performance of photographic film, television pickup tubes and the human eye. *J. Soc. Motion Pict. Eng.* **47,** 273–294.

Schade, O. (1956). Optical and photoelectric analog of the eye. *J. Opt. Soc. Am.* **46,** 721–739.

Sharp, P. and Mallard, J. (1974). A proposed model for the visual detection of signals in radioisotope display images. *Phys. Med. Biol.* **19,** 348–361.

Sharp, P. F. and Mallard, J. R. (1976). The measurement of the performance of the display system of a radioisotope imaging device: the multi-element band display. *Br. J. Radiol.* **49,** 270–277.

Sharp, P. F. and Marshall, I. (1981). The usefulness of indices measuring gamma-camera non-uniformity. *Phys. Med. Biol.* **26,** 149–153.

Sharp, P. F., Chesser, R. B. and Mallard, J. R. (1982). The influence of picture element size on the quality of clinical radionuclide images. *Phys. Med. Biol.* **27,** 913–926.

Swets, J. A., Tanner, W. P. and Birdsall, T. G. (1961). Decision processes in perception. *Psychol. Rev.* **68,** 301–340.

Starr, S. J., Metz, C. E., Lusted, L. B. and Goodenough, D. J. (1975). Visual detection and localization of radiographic images. *Radiology* **116,** 533–538.

Todd-Pokropek, A. E. and Pizer, S. M. (1977). Displays in scintigraphy. *In* "Medical Radionuclide Imaging", Vol. 1, pp. 505–536. IAEA, Vienna.

Tsui, B. W., Beck, R. N., Doi, K. and Metz, C. E. (1981). Analysis of recorded noise in nuclear medicine. *Phys. Med. Biol.* **26,** 883–902.

Wagner, R. F. and Weaver, K. E. (1973). An assortment of image quality indices for radiographic film-screen combinations. . . Can they be resolved? *Proc. Soc. Photo-Opt. Instrum. Eng.* **35,** 83–94.

Chapter 8

Data Analysis

8.1 Introduction

Computerised data processing is widely accepted as an integral part of the gamma-camera imaging system. Indeed in many cases this facility actually forms part of the camera, carrying out functions such as the display originally performed by analogue circuitry. In this chapter the emphasis will be on the use of data processing systems in clinical practice rather than on the hardware, details of which can be found in Erickson and Rollo (1983), for example.

Two main areas of application can be identified. First the processing system can be used to quantify the distribution of radiopharmaceutical. This facility is required most frequently for the analysis and presentation of data acquired in a dynamic study, in particular to reduce the large amount of data to more manageable proportions. It can also be used to quantify the absolute amount of radiopharmaceutical in an organ.

Secondly, image presentation can be manipulated either to vary the way in which data are displayed or to modify the original image data, prior to display, by using filtering algorithms. Only the latter will be dealt with in this chapter, display having been considered in Chapter 7.

8.2 Data reduction

Dynamic studies, such as renography, pose particular problems of presentation since not only must the spatial distribution of the radio-pharmaceutical be considered, but also temporal changes in that distribution. An examination of individual image frames is often effective for drawing the operator's attention to aspects of the study which may require further detailed analysis. The ciné mode display is particularly useful in this respect, the images being displayed rapidly in a continuous single-loop sequence.

One of the most useful features of the dynamic study is that changes in the amount of radiopharmaceutical present in different parts of the image can be measured quantitatively. Time–activity curves produced from user defined regions of interest (ROI) are the simplest way of achieving this and will be discussed in the next section. The value of the information obtained from these curves can be enhanced in some instances by the use of edge detection algorithms to define organ boundaries (Section 8.2.2). A further refinement of time–activity curve data can often be made by the application of deconvolution analysis (Section 8.2.3).

Time–activity curves produced from relatively large ROIs necessitate a loss in the quality of spatial information in the study, as the curve describes only the average behaviour of the radiopharmaceutical in that area of the organ encompassed by the ROI. Reducing the size of the ROI, and consequently using many ROIs to cover the organ, improves the spatial data but results in a larger number of curves. Functional or parametric imaging (Section 8.2.4) offers one solution to this problem.

8.2.1 Time–activity curves

One of the earliest methods for performing a quantitative dynamic study was to place scintillation probes over the areas of interest and record the output count rate on a chart recorder. Such studies depended for their success on correct positioning of the probe detectors prior to injection of the radiopharmaceutical.

By using a gamma camera instead of probes, the dynamic study can be recorded on the data proceessing system and analysed after the study has been completed. With modern large-field-of-view cameras there is little difficulty in ensuring that the organ is correctly positioned relative to the detector. The ROI from which the curve is to be generated can then be defined on an appropriate frame of the study using a light pen, joy-stick or keyboard controlled marker to delineate the region (Fig. 8.1a). Typically up to 16 ROIs can be drawn on a single study. For each image frame the counts in all pixels within an ROI are summed. The resulting plot of total counts (proportional to the activity) against time into the study is known as the time–activity curve (Fig. 8.1b).

Radionuclide Imaging Techniques

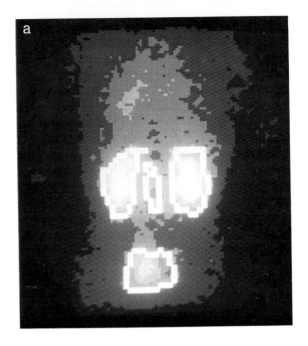

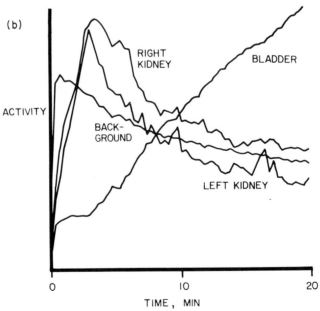

FIG. 8.1. (a) Regions of interest drawn around kidneys and bladder shown on one frame of a dynamic renal study. A background area is taken between the kidneys. (b) Time–activity curves produced from the regions of interest.

To give a more precise measure of the activity present in the organ, these curves can be corrected for background activity originating from overlying and underlying tissue.

In its simplest form, this background correction consists of using the data from a second ROI adjacent to or surrounding the first. In cases where the background is not uniform, more sophisticated methods have been applied. For example, in the technique proposed by Goris and colleagues (1976), the contribution $B(X,Y)$ of the background to the counts $C(X, Y)$ in element (X, Y) inside the ROI is given by bilinear interpolation

$$B(X, Y) = (B_1 + B_2)/2 \qquad (8.1)$$

where

$$B_1 = C(X, y_1) + [C(X, y_2) - C(X, y_1)][(Y - y_1)/(y_2 - y_1)] \quad (8.2)$$

and

$$B_2 = C(x_1, Y) + [C(x_2, Y) - C(x_1, Y)][(X - x_1)/(x_2 - x_1)] \qquad (8.3)$$

where (x_1, y_1) and (x_2, y_2) are the coordinates of the diagonally opposite vertices of a rectangular background ROI around the object.

8.2.2 Edge detection algorithms

The value of the information which can be extracted from a time–activity curve depends upon the accuracy with which the ROI can be delineated. Poor spatial resolution combined with organ motion inevitably leads to difficulties in defining the edge of an organ. Edge detection algorithms are attractive in that they offer a standard method for defining an edge and so remove variability often encountered when purely manual methods are employed. Secondly, in a cardiac study, it may be necessary to define the left ventricular border in perhaps 30 images acquired at different stages in the cardiac cycle. An automatic edge detection routine will, at the least, reduce this task.

The simplest approach is to apply a threshold to the image whereby all pixels having a value less than the threshold are set to zero, all those above to unity. While this may constitute a useful form of processing prior to manual delineation of the edge, it is not very efficient, particularly as the background cannot be assumed to be uniform.

Image filtering (see Section 8.3) is a second possibility, the ideal filter being one which enhances the high spatial frequencies associated with edges. In practice, an upper limit to the filter must be used to avoid undue emphasis on noise.

The third, and perhaps most frequently employed, method is differentiation of the image. This process can be considered as having three stages. First, the image is processed with a set of functions selected to emphasise features associated with edges; these processed images are then combined in the second stage to give the edge enhanced array. The third and final step is to make a decision about which of these elements constitute the edge. This state is common to other techniques, is perhaps the most difficult to automate and will usually require *a priori* knowledge of outline shape.

The simplest operator is one giving the first derivative. In a Cartesian coordinate system this can be simplified to

$$\Delta f_x = f(x,y) - f(x+1,y) \tag{8.4}$$

$$\Delta f_y = f(x,y) - f(x,y+1) \tag{8.5}$$

These two differentiated images must then be combined to emphasise the edge, whatever its orientation, with equal sensitivity. The most general combination function is the gradient defined as

$$[\Delta f_x^2 + \Delta f_y^2]^{1/2} \tag{8.6}$$

To save computational time, it can be approximated by

$$|\Delta f_x| + |\Delta f_y| \tag{8.7}$$

or maximum of

$$(|\Delta f_x|, |\Delta f_y|) \tag{8.8}$$

Rather than simply calculating the gradient from pairs of points, the average pixel value of those points on either side of the point in question can be taken, i.e.,

$$\frac{1}{N}\sum_{i=n-1}^{N} f(x,y+i) - \frac{1}{N}\sum_{i=n-1}^{N} f(x,y-i) \tag{8.9}$$

The size of this neighbourhood must be a compromise between the need to minimise noise (large value of N) and maintain spatial resolution (small N).

The second derivative can also be used. It is normally applied in the form of the Laplacian $(\partial^2 f/\partial x^2) + (\partial^2 f/\partial y^2)$ although Chang *et al.* (1980) have reported that it is unsatisfactory for nuclear medicine images, favouring lines and points over edges.

An extension of using the neighbourhood points is to attempt to fit a surface to these points. Using the minimum least-squares criterion, an $(N-1)$th degree polynomical can be fitted to an $N \times N$ neighbourhood array. Effectively the fitted surface produces a smoothed image. Having obtained this theoretical surface, the gradient and Laplacian can be calculated from it. In practice, for a given neighbourhood size, convolution operators can be applied directly to the image to give an output showing the smoothed image and Laplacian.

Once an enhanced edge image has been produced, it is then necessary to select those pixels constituting edges. In the case of Laplacian operators, enhanced values close to zero are indicative of edges, and, thus, a thresholding can be applied to leave only valid edge elements. In order to produce a continuous edge, such as would be needed to define an ROI, a tracking technique may be necessary. Other authors have used a minimal cost path approach in which the inverse values of the second derivative are taken as indicative of the cost of including a particular pixel in the boundary. The optimal boundary is that requiring the minimal cost to proceed from some beginning to the end point (Rosenfeld and Kak, 1976).

8.2.3 Deconvolution

The time–activity curve shows how the amount of radiopharmaceutical in an ROI drawn over an organ varies with time, the implicit assumption being that this curve also reflects the way in which the radiopharmaceutical is handled by the organ and hence organ function. The shape of the time–activity curve, however, depends not only upon the rate at which the radiopharmaceutical is handled by the organ but also on the rate at which it arrives at the organ.

The efficiency with which the organ handles the radiopharmaceutical can be measured by the time taken for the material to leave the organ. This so-called transit time will often not be a single value but a range of values reflecting the fact that the organ consists of many differently functioning cells or subcompartments. The resulting transit time spectrum $T(t)$ is the probability density function of the time taken for the radiopharmaceutical to move from organ input to output.

If all the radiopharmaceutical arrives at the organ simultaneously, then the time–activity curve will show only organ function, but in practice the material is injected into a peripheral vein and so may undergo mixing with a large volume of blood in its passage through heart and lungs.

Thus, although the volume of injected material may be very small, a fraction of a millilitre, it will have been diluted into a much larger volume before reaching the organ and an appreciable time may elapse before all the material has been presented to the organ.

If $I(t)$ represents the input time–activity curves of the radio-pharmaceutical and $O(t)$ the output from the organ, then

$$O(t) = \int_0^t T(s)I(t-s)\,ds \qquad (8.10)$$

i.e., the output time–activity curve is given by the input curve convolved with the transit time spectrum. The transit time spectrum is thus equivalent to an organ transfer function.

Time–activity curves as measured from a dynamic study do not show organ output $O(t)$ but rather the amount of material retained by the organ. This organ retention function $R(t)$ can be defined as

$$R(t) = 1 - \int_0^t T(s) \, ds \qquad (8.11)$$

and the time–activity curve $A(t)$ over the organ is therefore,

$$A(t) = \int_0^t R(s)I(t-s) \, ds \qquad (8.12)$$

The transit time spectrum can be derived from $R(t)$ since

$$T(t) = -(d/dt)R(t) \qquad (8.13)$$

To obtain $R(t)$ from the measured $A(t)$ it is necessary to deconvolve with the input function. In practice, noise on the time–activity curves will limit what can be achieved; this point will be considered again later. While deconvolution can be done by Laplace analysis (Kenny *et al.*, 1975), it does require that $I(t)$ be described analytically, so matrix inversion (Reeve and Crawley, 1974; Diffey *et al.*, 1976) which uses the experimentally measured form of $I(t)$ is generally preferred.

Equation (8.12) can be written in a discrete form as

$$A(t) = \sum_{s=0}^t R(s)I(t-s) \, \Delta s \qquad (8.14)$$

which can be expanded as a set of simultaneous equations:

$$A(0) = R(0)I(0) \, \Delta s$$
$$A(1) = R(1)I(0) \, \Delta s + R(0)I(1) \, \Delta s$$
$$A(n) = R(n)I(0) \, \Delta s + R(n-1)I(1) \, \Delta s + \cdots + R(0)I(n) \, \Delta s \quad (8.15)$$

and solving for R gives

$$R(0) = \frac{A(0)}{I(0) \, \Delta s}$$

$$R(1) = \frac{A(1)}{I(0) \, \Delta s} - \frac{R(0)I(1)}{I(0)}$$

$$R(n) = \frac{A(n)}{I(0) \, \Delta s} - \frac{R(n-1)I(1)}{I(0)} - \cdots - \frac{R(0)I(n)}{I(0)} \qquad (8.16)$$

Or writing Eq. (8.12) in matrix form

$$\mathbf{A} = \mathbf{R} \cdot \mathbf{I} \Delta s \qquad (8.17)$$

and so

$$R = \mathbf{A} \cdot \mathbf{I}^{-1} / \Delta s \qquad (8.18)$$

where I^{-1} is the inverted I, which since I is triangular is simple to perform.

Rather than displaying the complete transit time spectrum, there are obvious advantages in describing it by a small number of indices. The one most commonly used is the mean transit time $\bar{t}$. This can be derived directly from $R(t)$, avoiding the need for differentiation, since

$$\bar{t} = \int_0^\infty t T(t)\, dt \bigg/ \int_0^\infty T(t)\, dt = \int_0^\infty R(t)\, dt \bigg/ R(0) \qquad (8.19)$$

The inverse of $\bar{t}$ can be shown to be equal to the blood flow per unit volume to the organ (Zierler, 1965).

Other indices which have been used (Piepsz et al., 1982) include

(i) $T20$, the time taken for $R(t)$ to fall to 20% of its initial value
(ii) $T80$, the time for $R(t)$ to fall to 80% of its initial value
(iii) $R(0)$, the initial height of $R(t)$.

Deconvolution analysis has been used with several types of clinical studies such as cerebral blood flow (Britton et al., 1980) and in cardiac work (Alderson et al., 1979; Ham et al., 1981) but is most frequently applied to renal imaging (Reeve and Crawley, 1974; Kenny et al., 1975; Diffey et al., 1976; Piepsz et al., 1982).

To conclude this discussion of deconvolution, an example of its practical application to renography will be given. The first consideration is to ensure that the time–activity curves represent only activity originating from renal tissue. A background correction (Section 8.2.1) must be made using an ROI drawn between the two kidneys but avoiding major blood pools (Fig. 8.2a). Also the renal pelvis must be excluded from the kidney ROI if the transit times are to reflect renal tissue alone. This can be done by producing a functional image (see Section 8.2) showing the time of maximum activity for each image pixel. The values for renal pelvis will be much greater than for renal tissue, as demonstrated in Fig. 8.2b.

As has been mentioned already, the success of deconvolution depends upon noise being kept to a minimum. Data bounding (Diffey and Corfield, 1976) and cubic spline fitting (Fleming and Kenny, 1977) have been used to smooth the data in the time–activity curve. Obviously a compromise must be reached between reducing noise and distorting the curve. In Fig. 8.2c smoothing has been carried out with a simple five-point filter of values (1, 2, 4, 2, 1), applied four times to the curve.

The choice of a suitable area in the image from which to measure $I(t)$ is also a problem. In this example $I(t)$ has been taken from an ROI drawn

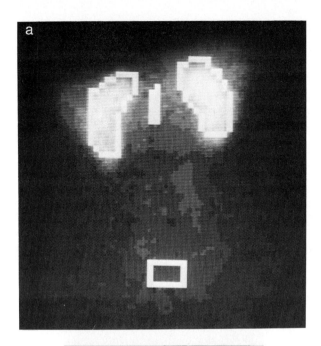

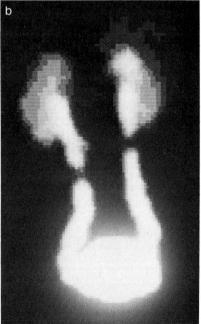

FIG. 8.2. (a) Regions of interest around the kidneys and the bladder. The small region of interest between the kidneys is taken as the background. (b) Functional image of the time at which the counts in a pixel reach a maximum. Those pixels in the kidneys representing the renal pelvis have the highest values. (c) Smoothed time activity curves for renal tissue, bladder and the area taken as the input function. (d) The retention functions for right and left kidneys, the thicker line showing the final version of the function after the vascular component has been subtracted. (Courtesy of Dr. H. Gemmell, University of Aberdeen.)

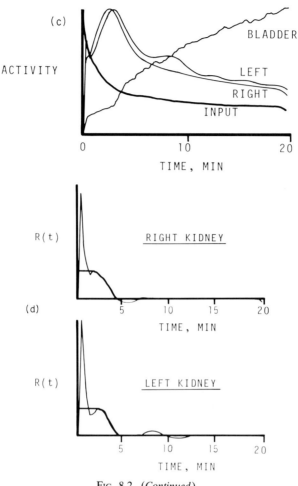

FIG. 8.2. (*Continued*)

over the heart; other authors have used the liver or, in the case of a transplanted kidney, the descending aorta.

The deconvolved retention function $R(t)$ is itself noisy and before further analysis it is smoothed once by the same filter as used on the curve and truncated when it first becomes negative (Fig. 8.2d). The final function shows a rapid initial fall, attributable to vascular outflow of material (Reeve and Crawley, 1974). The exact shape of the vascular function is very sensitive to choice of $I(t)$ and the background subtraction used: although of potential use in detecting renal artery stenosis, it is, in general, of little interest and, as shown in Fig. 8.2d, is subtracted from the final retention function. The renal retention function is the succeeding, slowly varying, function.

In this example $\bar{t}$ is 211 sec for the left kidney and 196 sec for the right. The renogram curves of Fig. 8.3a show reduced function and poor drainage from the left kidney. This is reflected in the retention function (Fig. 8.3b), which indicates that $\bar{t}$ is 671 sec for the left kidney compared with 259 sec for the right one.

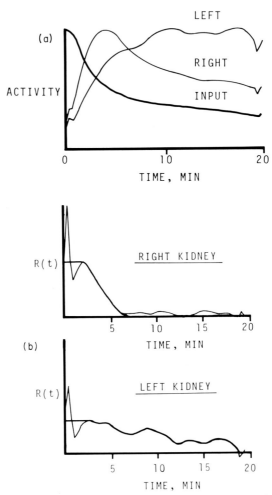

FIG. 8.3. (a) Renogram curves showing reduced function and poor drainage from the left kidney and a normal right kidney. (b) The retention function for the left kidney is considerably broader than that for the right one. (Courtery of Dr. H. Gemmell, University of Aberdeen.)

The value of deconvolution analysis is somewhat reduced by the substantial smoothing used to reduce noise to an acceptable level. This not only raises the possibility that subtle features of the time–activity curves might be lost, but since various centres use different smoothing techniques, a comparison of results is difficult.

8.2.4 Functional imaging

While time-activity curves provide a simple way of demonstrating temporal changes in radiopharmaceutical distribution, they do so at the expense of spatial information. Only by using a large number of small ROIs can spatial information be restored, but this not only will lead to noisy curves but also will introduce the problem of how to display all the curves in an easily understandable form.

One way of avoiding this problem is to describe the time–activity curve by a small number of indices. By displaying the index value at the same spatial position as the ROI used to produce the curve, functional images can be created. The dynamic study is thus reduced to a small number of images each showing the spatial distribution of the values of one particular index.

The choice of indices is a major problem particularly as they must be insensitive to noise in the curves. In an ideal case each index would reflect one aspect of the physiology of the organ under study, but rarely is sufficient knowledge of the behaviour of the radiopharmaceutical available to do this, and in practice the indices simply reflect the shape of the time–activity curve.

As an example of how functional images can be produced, consider the method used by Băsić and colleagues (1983) to describe a cholescintigraphic study. In cholescintigraphy (Ronai *et al.*, 1975) the radiopharmaceutical is removed from the blood stream by the polygonal cells of the liver, draining through the hepatic ducts and biliary ducts and into gall bladder or duodenum (see Fig. 2.15). A poorly functioning liver will show a generally slow passage of material to the hepatic ducts, while an obstruction such as a gall stone will delay or completely block the movement of material (Clarke *et al.*, 1982). It is particularly easy to produce functional images in this study since the radiopharmaceutical readily concentrates in the normal liver giving a high count density image with relatively little statistical noise on the time–activity curves.

Băsić chose four indices to describe the normal time–activity curve from an ROI over the liver (Fig. 8.4), the slope at 4 min post-injection of the second-degree polynomical fitted to phase 1 (S_1), the slopes of the best straight lines fitted to phases 2 and 3 (S_2 and S_3), and the time t_{max} at which the curve peaks.

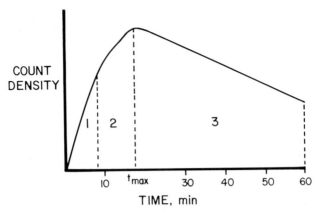

Fig. 8.4. Average time-activity curve for normal liver tissue.

The first three indices are of little use on their own as their values depend upon the absolute count density which, in turn, will depend not only upon the function per unit mass of hepatic tissue but also on the thickness of tissue in that area of the liver associated with the ROI. This will have an effect on the functional image as liver thickness can vary considerably, being greatest over the right lobe. In order to eradicate this

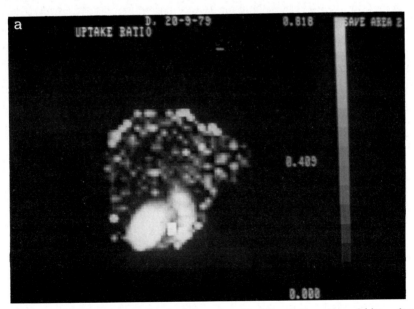

Fig. 8.5. Functional images showing (a) uptake ratio, (b) excretion ratio and (c) t_{max} for a normal study.

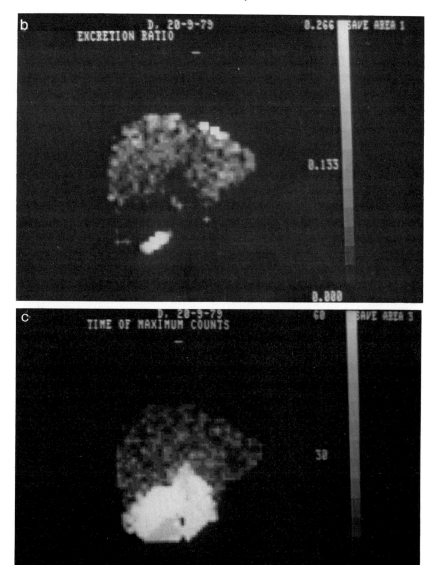

FIG. 8.5. (*Continued*)

effect the ratios S_2/S_1 (the uptake ratio) and S_3/S_1 (the excretion ratio) were taken, together with t_{max}, as the final indices.

In the normal patient (Fig. 8.5), the values of the uptake ratio, excretion ratio and t_{max} are uniform throughout the liver. As material is continuously draining through the common bile duct and into the gall bladder, these areas have an elevated uptake ratio, no excretion and a t_{max} value which is effectively equal to the length of the study. When there is an obstruction, such as a gall stone, preventing the radiopharmaceutical from leaving the liver (Fig. 8.6), there is no excretion over most of the liver, an elevated t_{max}, but the uptake ratio is largely unaffected.

The most common application of functional imaging is to describe the clearance of radioactive gas, such as 133-xenon, from the lungs. The patient breathes a mixture of air and radioactive xenon from a closed breathing system for about 100 sec until it has had time to equilibrate in the lungs. The circuit is then switched so that the patient breathes air alone, the expired xenon being trapped in a filter. The whole investigation is recorded as a dynamic study, the patient sitting with the back against the gamma camera.

The resulting time–activity curve over the lungs can be divided into three sections showing wash-in of gas, equilibrium and wash-out. The parameter of clinical interest is the rate of clearance of gas from the lungs.

The simplest index that can be chosen is the time constant of the wash-out phase, but the validity of this choice does depend on the assumption that this part of the study is adequately described by a

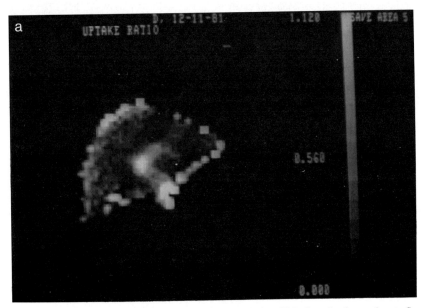

FIG. 8.6. Functional images as in Fig. 5 for a study in which there is obstruction to flow through the common bile duct.

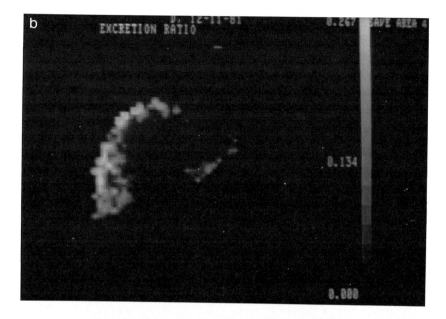

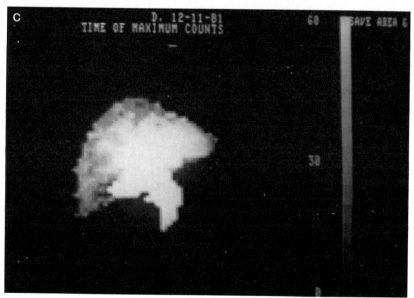

FIG. 8.6. (*Continued*)

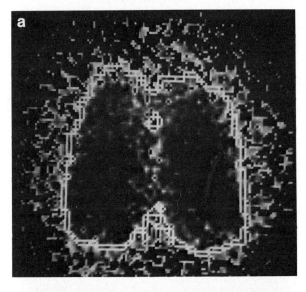

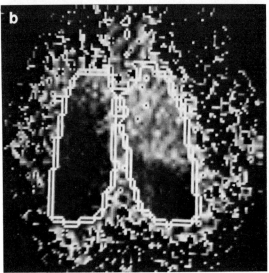

FIG. 8.7. Ventilation perfusion ratio (V/Q) images for (a) a normal patient and (b) one with emphysema. Both images are the posterior view and lung outlines are shown.

mono-exponential curve. Instead it is more usual, and indeed simpler, to calculate the mean transit time $\bar{t}$ of the gas. It can be shown (Zierler, 1965) that $\bar{t}$ is simply given by

$$\text{area under wash-out curve/equilibrium count rate} \qquad (8.20)$$

The denominator acts as a normalisation factor for the total lung volume, and $\bar{t}$ is equal to the ratio of lung volume to air flow.

Figure 8.7 shows a pair of these so-called V/Q images. The normal patient shows uniform V/Q ratio throughout both lungs, while the patient with emphysema has a high V/Q ratio in the upper lobes of the right lung, and to a lesser extent in the left one, demonstrating slow gas wash-out, i.e., long transit time.

Another interesting application of functional imaging is in cardiac investigations. By labelling the blood pool with a radioactive tracer such as 99m-Tc-labelled human serum albumin, the cardiac chambers can be clearly visualised. It is of clinical interest to view the changes in the shape and volume of the left ventricle during the cardiac cycle. As insufficient counts would be acquired during the cardiac cycle, it is necessary to collect counts over several hundred cycles. To ensure that each image in the dynamic study always receives counts from the same part of the cardiac cycle, i.e., to keep the different cycles 'in phase', it is necessary to synchronise data acquisition with a signal from an electrocardiograph attached to the patient (Fig. 8.8). From this set of consecutive images throughout the cardiac cycle, the time–activity curve over the left ventricle (Fig. 8.9) can be measured to show the change in ventricular blood volume during the average cardiac cycle.

It has been suggested (Bossuyt *et al.*, 1980) that this curve can be described by a sine (or cosine function) or, more specifically, by the first harmonic of the Fourier series of the curve, i.e., the counts in the ROI at

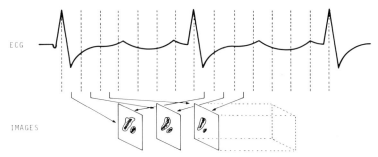

Fig. 8.8. Gated cardiac study. Data is entered into the first frame of the dynamic study when the R wave of each cycle is detected. The duration of each frame is present before the study starts.

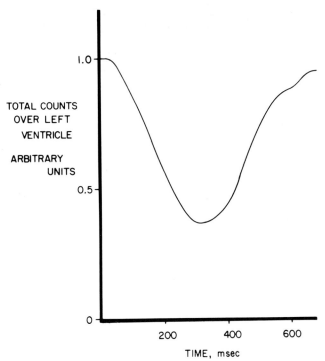

Fɪɢ. 8.9 Time–activity curve over the left ventricle in a normal patient.

time t is given by

$$C(t) = a + b \sin(2\pi ft + \phi) \qquad (8.21)$$

where f is the reciprocal of the number of frames per cardiac cycle.

The values of b for the time–activity curves generated from each pixel can be used to form the 'amplitude' image showing areas of similar count rate. This image may be useful for defining the edge of the ventricle. The functional image of ϕ, the 'phase' image, shows areas which start contracting at the same time (Fig. 8.10).

Houston and colleagues (1982) have criticised the assumption that the sine function adequately describes the shape of the left ventricle curve and suggest an approach using a more general function based on principal component analysis.

8.2.5   Principal component analysis

As mentioned in the previous section, the choice of indices for functional images is frequently based on the shape of a curve for a normal study and is

Radionuclide Imaging
Techniques

PETER F. SHARP

Department of Bio-Medical Physics and Bio-Engineering
University of Aberdeen
Aberdeen, Scotland

PHILIP P. DENDY

Department of Medical Physics
Addenbrookes Hospital
Cambridge, England

W. IAN KEYES

Department of Medical Physics
Cumberland Infirmary
Carlisle, Cumbria, England

 1985

ACADEMIC PRESS, INC.

Harcourt Brace Jovanovich, Publishers
London   Orlando   San Diego   New York
Austin   Montreal   Sydney   Tokyo   Toronto

ACADEMIC PRESS INC. (LONDON) LTD.
24–28 Oval Road
LONDON NW1 7DX

United States Edition published by
ACADEMIC PRESS, INC.
Orlando, Florida 32887

British Library Cataloguing in Publication Data

Sharp, Peter F.
    Radionuclide imaging techniques.–(Medical
    physics series)
    1. Imaging systems in medicine   2. Diagnosis
    I. Title   II. Dendy, P.P.   III. Keyes, W. Ian
    IV. Series
    616.07'54   R857.06

Library of Congress Cataloging in Publication Data

Sharp, Peter F.
    Radionuclide imaging techniques.

    (Medical physics series)
    Bibliography: p.
    Includes index.
    1. Radioisotope scanning.   2. Imaging systems in
medicine.   I. Dendy, P. P.   II. Keyes, W. Ian.   III. Title.
IV. Series.
RC78.7.R4S5   1985   616.07'575   85-5267
ISBN 0–12–639020–7 (alk. paper)
ISBN 0–12–639021–5 (paperback)

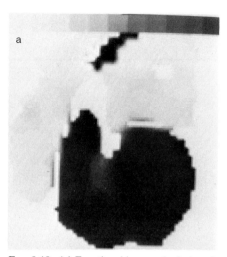
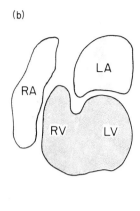

F$_{IG}$. 8.10. (a) Functional image of relative phases of the time–activity curves in different regions of the heart. (b) Outlines of right and left ventricles and atria as they appear in (a). (Courtesy of the Departments of Nuclear Medicine and Medical Physics, Addenbrookes Hospital, Cambridge and the Regional Cardiac Unit, Papworth Hospital, Cambs.).

further constrained by the need to use analytic functions. These factors, combined with the necessity to produce only a small number of indices, make it almost inevitable that only the grossest features of the curve can be adequately represented.

Principal component analysis has been used by several workers as a way of overcoming these problems. Using a sample of typical time–activity curves, this approach extracts features, or principal components, common to all the curves. These components are themselves curves with the same number of data points as the original time–activity curves.

A particular time–activity curve can then be formed by summing the principal component curves after each one has been weighted by an appropriate factor. This method has obvious similarities to the Fourier transform, but while the Fourier transform is based on sine and cosine functions, no such restriction is placed on the shape of the principal components. A full description of the technique is given by Andrews (1972).

The particular value of principal component analysis to functional imaging is that the components can be ranked into an order reflecting the amount of information they provide about curve shape. It is frequently found that only a small number of components (and their weighting factors) are needed to give a close approximation to the original curves.

Since the principal components are common to all time–activity curves for the study in question, the weighting factors alone can be used to create functional images. Schmidlin (1979) has used this idea to analyse reno-grams, only three factors being found necessary. The physiological relevance of such factors is questionable, although Schmidlin suggests that each functional image shows areas of the organ of similar, if unspecified, function.

Barber *et al.*, (1974) have analysed the curves of a gastric-emptying study using seven factors. Applying multi-variate analysis to the factors, they showed that the factors permitted a better discrimination between pathological conditions than could be obtained from simpler analytic functions. Houston and MacLeod (1980), however, came to the conclusion that if the handling of the radiopharmaceutical could be described adequately in terms of a simple compartmental system then there was little to be gained by principal component analysis.

Oppenheim and Appledorn (1980) used principal component analysis as an aid to producing conventional functional images. They calculated the principal components from the group of time–activity curves and selected the most important ones, i.e:, those carrying the most information. If a particular curve is then constructed using these chief components and appropriate weighting factors, a relatively noiseless version of the curve will be produced. The values of the indices for the functional images can then be easily derived from these 'smoothed' curves.

Principal component analysis is not confined to time–activity curves: it can also be applied to images if they are first reduced to simple one-dimensional vectors. Barber (1976) proposed that a 'typical' normal brain image could be derived by extracting the principal components from a group of clinically normal images. In his study only 10 components were necessary to account for most of the features in a set of lateral views. When analysing a suspected abnormal image, the weighting factors corresponding to these 'normal' components are first calculated and an image is reconstructed. This image will show the normal features of the image under consideration and if subtracted from the original image should expose any abnormal features. Barber suggested that the statistical significance of these features could be evaluated or alternatively the features emphasised before adding them back into the original image (Fig. 8.11).

This work has been extended to studies of brain blood flow (Barber, 1980) and liver function (Barber and Nijran, 1981), while Bazin and colleagues (1980) have also applied it to thyroid imaging.

The main problem with principal component analysis is in producing the principal components. For effective application of the analysis the images used must be standardised; in particular they should be of the same size and orientation. This is a particular problem with liver images where organ shape can vary considerably.

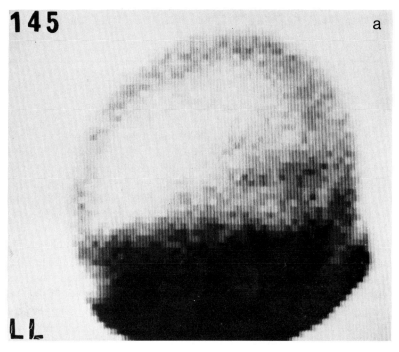

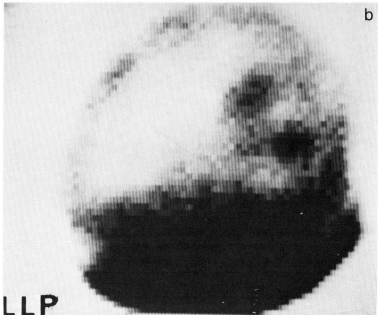

FIG. 8.11. A lateral view of a brain scan (a) before and (b) after processing with a principal components technique. The abnormality in the occipital region is clearly seen after processing. [From Barber (1976).]

The calculation of the principal components requires a relatively large amount of computation and will often need a larger computer than that available in most nuclear medicine departments at present. Also, to facilitate this process, the images must be coarsely digitised—for example, Barber (1980) used only a 24×16 matrix for brain images—and this limits the sensitivity of the technique for detecting small features.

8.2.6 Quantification of radionuclide uptake

In many clinical situations the ability to measure precisely the amount of radiopharmaceutical concentrating in an organ or tumour would greatly enhance the diagnostic information. Ideally this quantitative information would be derived directly from the image count density allowing the measurement to be made over some precisely defined area. The use of tomographic devices for this purpose has been discussed in Chapter 4. In this section we will examine how such information might be obtained from conventional plane views.

Both the rectilinear scanner and gamma camera can be used to give quantitative information, but, in general, to produce an absolute measure of radiopharmaceutical concentration it is necessary to supplement the image count density with additional measurements. As discussed in Section 3.4, whole body counters are frequently used for quantitative work, even with very low levels of activity, but they have extremely limited imaging capabilities.

Three factors must be considered when quantifying data.

(i)   the response $D(x, y, z)$ of the detecting device as a function both of the source–detector distance z and position in the plane (x, y) parallel to the detector

(ii)   the effect of attenuation and scatter of emitted radiation by overlying tissue

(iii)   the reproducibility in performance of imaging device and radio-pharmaceutical.

As an initial approximation, let us assume that the detector response $D(x, y, z)$ is invariant in the plane (x, y) depending only on the source–detector distance z. This assumption is reasonable for the rectilinear scanner, most types of whole body counters and, to a lesser extent, the gamma camera.

Figure 8.12a shows the simplest form of the problem, a thin object of activity A per unit volume situated at a depth a in medium of linear attenuation coefficient μ and total thickness T. Attenuation is assumed to

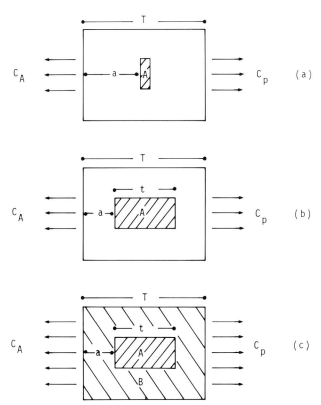

FIG. 8.12. (a) A thin object having activity A per unit volume at a depth a in a non-active volume of thickness T whose linear attenuation coefficient is μ. (b) As in (a) but the source thickness t is now not negligible. The linear attenuation coefficient of the source is assumed to be μ. (c) As in (b) but the background material surrounding the source now has activity B per unit volume.

be exponential, an approximation which may not be valid when there is appreciable scatter present. The detector over the anterior surface will record a count rate

$$C_A = D(a)\,A e^{-\mu a} \tag{8.22}$$

while at the posterior surface the count rate is

$$C_P = D(T-a)\,A e^{-\mu(T-a)} \tag{8.23}$$

The geometric mean of these two count rates is

$$\sqrt{C_A C_P} = [D(a)\,D(T-a)]^{1/2}\,e^{-\mu T/2} \tag{8.24}$$

For a rectilinear scanner with a focussed collimator and a gamma camera with a parallel-hole collimator, D is independent of z, hence

$$\sqrt{C_A C_P} = D e^{-\mu T/2} \tag{8.25}$$

The geometric mean of anterior and posterior count rates is independent of source depth, the only additional measurement needed being body thickness T.

For several types of whole body counters D varies exponentially with depth (Sorenson, 1974). Assuming

$$D = D(0)e^{-kz} \tag{8.26}$$

then

$$\sqrt{C_A C_P} = D(0)\, e^{-(k+\mu)T/2} \tag{8.27}$$

and again the result is dependent only on body thickness.

The body thickness can be estimated by external measurement with calipers but this may prove inaccurate in the case of an irregular body. An effective thickness can be obtained by transmission imaging. A plane source of radioactivity, preferably from a radionuclide identical to that under investigation, is placed beneath the patient, and the count rate I_T of the transmitted radiation is measured. The same measurement is made without the patient giving an unattenuated count rate I_0.

Then

$$I_T = I_0 e^{-\mu T} \tag{8.28}$$

so

$$T = (1/\mu)\, \ln(I_0/I_T) \tag{8.29}$$

Thus Eq. (8.25) can be written as

$$\sqrt{C_A C_P} = D(I_T/I_0)^{1/2} \tag{8.30}$$

If the thickness t of the source is not negligible (Fig. 8.12b), then self-attenuation of its radiation must now be considered. Thus, for a depth-independent detector

$$C_A = DA \int_{z=a}^{a+t} e^{-\mu z} dz \tag{8.31}$$

$$C_P = DA \int_{z=T-a-t}^{T-a} e^{-\mu z} dz \tag{8.32}$$

and

$$\sqrt{C_A C_P} = \frac{DA}{\mu/2} \sinh\left(\frac{\mu t}{2}\right) \exp(-\mu T/2) \tag{8.33}$$

Again the geometric mean provides a measure of A which is independent of source depth a, but now it is necessary to measure the thicknesses of both the body T and organ t. The latter is usually estimated from lateral views.

If the depth response of the detector is exponential, then

$$\sqrt{C_A C_P} = D\frac{A}{\mu/2}\sinh[(\mu + k)t/2]\exp(-\mu T/2) \qquad (8.34)$$

The model has been employed by Fleming (1979) to quantify liver uptake from gamma-camera images.

In the general form of the problem (Fig. 8.12c), there is activity B per unit volume in the background for which the attenuation coefficient is also μ. Then for the depth-independent collimator

$$C_A = [(A - B)/\mu]e^{-\mu a}[1 - e^{-\mu t}] + (B/\mu)(1 - e^{-\mu T}) \qquad (8.35)$$

and

$$C_P = [(A - B)/\mu]e^{\mu a}e^{-\mu(T-t)}(1 - e^{-\mu t}) + (B/\mu)(1 - e^{-\mu T}) \quad (8.36)$$

No further simplification is achieved by taking the geometric mean.

For the low-energy gamma rays used in imaging, it is impossible when using conventional detectors to discriminate against scattered radiation. Unfortunately, with the Compton process the amount of scatter is dependent upon the shape of source and background, and the use of a simple exponential function to describe attenuation will be inadequate. Fleming (1979) avoids this difficulty by using a liver-shaped phantom, surrounded with the appropriate amount of tissue-equivalent material, to measure how count rate varies with depth z. This measurement will, thus, include variations attributable to changes in both D and μ.

Ferrant and Cauwe (1979), also using gamma-camera data, proposed that a set of calibration factors should be produced for a range of source geometries. They conceded that such a procedure is 'tedious' since it would be necessary to carry out this calibration for each imaging device employed and whenever changes were made in pulse height analyser settings.

It is difficult to give an estimate of the accuracies of these techniques since accuracy will depend upon the complexity of the task and type of imaging equipment used. For whole-body counting systems a thorough discussion is to be found in Sorenson (1974). Ferrant and Cauwe (1979), who used the most detailed analysis, validated their approach by quantifying the amount of radioactivity in the stomach after ingestion of 18 MBq of sulphur colloid by volunteers. The results of nine measurements showed a 9.4% error. Fleming (1979) judged the error in his technique to be between 5 and 10%.

Pitt and Sharp (1981) looked at the errors involved in using a gamma camera for quantifying uptake but from the point of view of the reproducibility of the measurements rather than overall accuracy. They calculated the ratio of the activity in a small Perspex cube and the count rate calculated from its image, a quantity they called the activity calibration factor. For a source at a known and constant depth in a tissue-equivalent medium, the error in predicting activity from the number of counts within a region of interest drawn around the image varied from 5.9 to 11%. This was made up of a random component, caused by day-to-day variations in camera response and differences in sensitivity across the camera's field of view and a systematic error related to changes in source size. The latter component is presumably the effect of source size on the amount of Compton-scattered radiation included in the ROI and produces an average error of about 5%. Thus, irrespective of the formula used for obtaining the quantitative information, a minimum error of at least 6% was to be expected.

One final factor which must be considered is the reproducibility in the behaviour of the radiopharmaceutical. Unfortunately very little work appears to have been done on this subject.

8.3 Image filtering

Image filtering offers a great potential for improving image quality. Early attempts were limited to analogue data and involved such simple manipulations as noise blurring by defocussing the cathode ray tube beam. With the introduction of computer-interfaced processing systems in the mid-1970s, the sophistication of filtering techniques improved greatly. See, for example, Todd-Pokropek (1980) for a general review of the subject.

An image filter is most conveniently described by its effect on the spatial frequency content of an image. Typically, nuclear medicine images will only contain spatial frequencies up to about 1.5 cycles/cm (see Section 5.3). They also contain a large amount of statistical noise. These factors place a considerable constraint on what filtering can achieve.

Two main techniques are used for implementing the filter process: the Fourier transform method and the convolution method. In the former the image is first Fourier transformed into its spatial frequency components. Each of these components is multiplied by a weighting factor (the filter), and the inverse Fourier transform is applied to convert this filtered data back into an image in real space.

The convolution method, also known as the finite impulse response method, is the more commonly used technique. The function showing the variation of weighting factors with spatial frequency is transformed from frequency space into an array of weighting values in real space. These are then convolved with the image to give the final filtered image. This approach is illustrated in Fig. 8.13. The two techniques are described in detail by Miller and Sampathkumaran (1982). It is worth emphasising that these two techniques are equivalent, convolution in real space being identical to multiplication in frequency space. The difference lies in the method of application.

The major problem in filter design is not that of specifying what the filter should do, but rather achieving it within the restrictions on memory size and processing speed imposed by nuclear medicine computer systems. With the continuing development of computers and the introduction of array processors (King *et al.*, 1983), these restrictions are becoming less severe but nevertheless do pose a problem.

Figure 8.14a shows an ideal low-pass filter in the frequency domain, all spatial frequencies up to a maximum of 0.6 cycles/cm are transmitted unmodified by the filter while higher ones are excluded. When such a sharp edge is Fourier transformed into real space (Fig. 8.14b), many factors are required to represent it adequately. If, to reduce filtering time, we choose to use only a few of these factors, say the first six, then (Fig. 8.14a) the actual shape of the filter differs from the original. Thus, if the requirement is for the filter to have only a small number of factors, the choice of filter. shapes will be limited. This particular example shows that it will not be possible to produce a step filter, and one having a much less abrupt cut-off will be necessary.

A second problem is the oscillations seen at high frequencies. These are a result of the sudden truncation of the frequency series and will produce 'ringing' in the filtered image. They can be avoided by windowing the series, i.e., multiplying it with a function which weights the factors so that they steadily decrease to zero (Fig. 8.14a). Typical window functions are the Hamming, Hanning and Blackman (Blackman and Tukey, 1978). Most of the filters used on nuclear medicine images fall into one of three categories: smoothing, resolution recovery and enhancing.

8.3.1 Smoothing filters

These filters are used primarily for reducing noise, thereby increasing the signal to noise ratio (SNR). Since noise in nuclear medicine images is most evident at high spatial frequencies, these filters are designed to attenuate high frequencies while sparing low frequencies.

Figure 8.15a shows three smoothing filters, with different high-frequency cut-offs. As the cut-off is moved to lower frequencies noise is

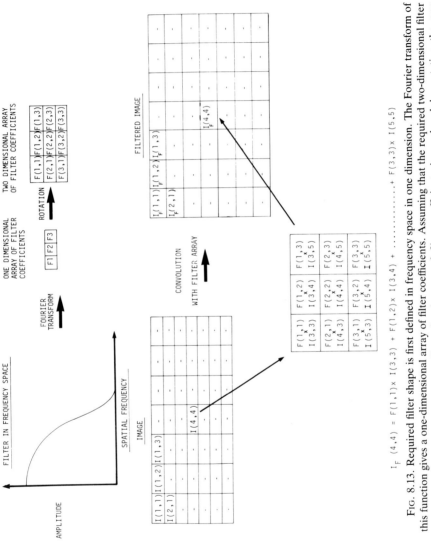

$$I_F(4,4) = F(1,1) \times I(3,3) + F(1,2) \times I(3,4) + \ldots \ldots \ldots + F(3,3) \times I(5,5)$$

FIG. 8.13. Required filter shape is first defined in frequency space in one dimension. The Fourier transform of this function gives a one-dimensional array of filter coefficients. Assuming that the required two-dimensional filter is circularly symmetrical, the two-dimensional array of filter coefficients is produced by rotating the one dimensional array. The image is then filtered by convolving it with this filter coefficient array. An example of how this is done is shown for image pixel $I(4, 4)$.

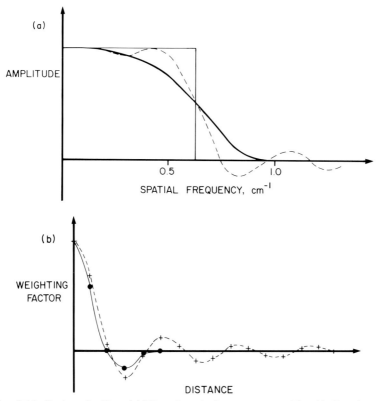

FIG. 8.14. Design of a filter. (a) Filter shape in frequency space. The thin line shows the shape of the ideal low-pass filter, the broken line the resulting shape if only six factors are used, and the thicker solid line the result of using a Hanning window on the factors. (b) Filter shape in real space. The dashed line is the shape of the ideal low-pass filter. The crosses show the weighting factors (filter coefficients) if the image array is assumed to be made up of 4-mm pixels. The solid line shows the weighting factors after a Hanning window has been used, the solid circles being the values of the weighting factor.

reduced but eventually image sharpness suffers as well (Fig.8.15b, c and d). One of the most frequently used smoothing filters in nuclear medicine is a nine-point array of weighting factors

$$\begin{matrix} 1 & 2 & 1 \\ 2 & 4 & 2 \\ 1 & 2 & 1 \end{matrix}$$

representing a pseudo-Gaussian filter shape.

Smoothing filters are of most value on images where the count density is low and, hence, noise is high. In many studies the count density, and hence

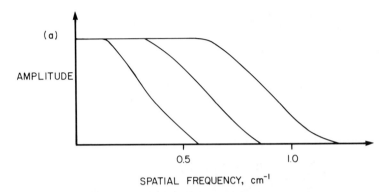

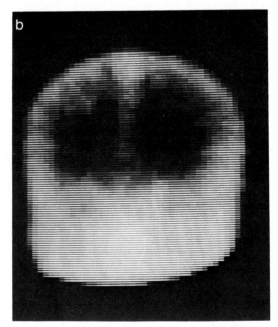

FIG. 8.15. (a) Three low-pass smoothing filters in frequency space. An anterior view brain image (Fig. 7.3) after processing with the filter with a cut-off frequency of (b) 1.4 cycles cm^{-1}, (c) 0.85 cycles cm^{-1} and (d) 0.6 cycles cm^{-1}.

the amount of smoothing required, will vary from one part of the image to another. Non-stationary filtering allows the degree of smoothing, or indeed the type of filter, to be varied according to the count density in that region of the image. Obviously such filtering can only be implemented with the convolution method.

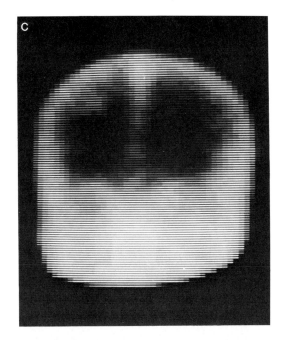

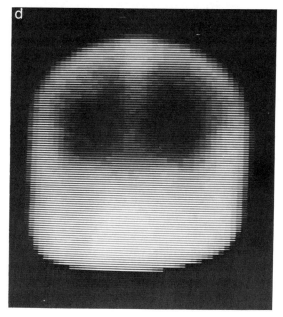

FIG. 8.15. (*Continued*)

Reducing the effect of noise may also be considered as a problem of maximising the SNR. This maximisation can be achieved by making the shape of the filter (in real space) identical to that of the feature to be detected (Tanaka and Iinuma, 1970). This 'matched filter', of course, necessitates *a priori* knowledge of feature shape. Also, while optimising the SNR it does so without any regard for correctly reproducing the shape of the feature.

8.3.2 Resolution recovery

As stated earlier, the degradation of spatial information by the imaging device is described by the system transfer function TF, the image I being the result of convolving the object O with the transfer function.

In frequency space convolution becomes multiplication, so

$$I(f_x, f_y) = O(f_x, f_y) \times \text{TF}(f_x, f_y) \tag{8.37}$$

Knowing TF it is theoretically possible to reconstruct the object by filtering the image with a function equal to the inverse of TF,

$$O(f_x, f_y) = I(f_x, f_y) \times \text{TF}^{-1}(f_x, f_y) \tag{8.38}$$

This is the principle of the refocussing or resolution recovery filter.

The general shape of a gamma-camera modulation transfer function (MTF) is one which falls rapidly at high frequencies; the simple resolution recovery filter will thus give greatest weight to these frequencies. This has the unfortunate consequence that noise will be amplified and so in a practical form this filter must be rolled off at some predetermined frequency (Fig. 8.16). For example, Tanaka and Iinuma (1970) proposed a filter of the form

$$\text{MTF}^{-1}(f_x, f_y) \qquad \text{for} \qquad f_x, f_y < f_c \tag{8.39}$$

and

$$\text{MTF}(f_x, f_y)/\text{MTF}(f_c, f_c)^2 \qquad \text{for} \qquad f_x, f_y > f_c \tag{8.40}$$

where the critical frequency $f_c = 0.45/\text{FWHM}$, FWHM being the full width at half-maximum height of the line or point spread function (PSF). Metz (1969) proposed a set of filters in which MTF^{-1} is expanded in a polynomial series of $(1 - \text{MTF}^2)$, so giving a filter of the form

$$[1 - (1 - \text{MTF}^2)^{n+1}]/\text{MTF} \tag{8.41}$$

This is a combination of a smoothing filter and a refocussing filter. For $n = 0$ it is the matched filter while when $n \to \infty$ it becomes the inverse filter.

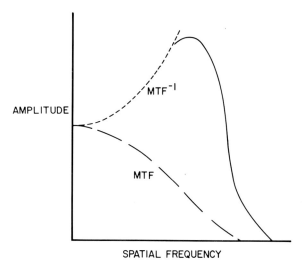

SPATIAL FREQUENCY

FIG. 8.16. Resolution recovery filter.

The refocussing problem has also been tackled using the maximum entropy technique. All possible images produced by randomly distributing intensity levels amongst image pixels are considered. Given an image and a knowledge of the errors associated with the data, then most of these possible images will be unrealistic representations and so can be disregarded. Of those that are judged consistent with the data, the most frequently occurring one is chosen as the best representation of the data. This image will be the most uniform one which is consistent with the image data.

According to Gull and Daniel (1978), the most convenient choice of statistic for testing consistency is the chi-squared statistic

$$\sum_k \frac{(I_k^P - I_k)^2}{\sigma_k^2} \tag{8.42}$$

where I_k^P is the intensity of the kth pixel in the postulated image and I_k that in the measured image and σ_k the standard deviation of the assumed Gaussian error associated with this measurement. The term I_k^P will, of course, be the convolution of the known PSF of the imaging device with the postulated object.

From the group of consistent solutions one must be selected as "best". This choice is made on the basis of the entropy of the image. Entropy has been defined in various ways; that used by Frieden (1972) and adopted by Gull and Daniell (1978) is

$$-\sum I_k^{PN} \log I_k^{PN} \tag{8.43}$$

where

$$I_k^{PN} = I_k^P \bigg/ \sum_k I_k^P \qquad (8.44)$$

i.e., the normalised image intensity. The most probable image is that which maximises the entropy.

As well as being used for deconvolving plane views, this has also been applied to tomographic reconstructions (Kemp, 1981). While undoubtedly producing images which are freer from artefacts than other methods, the maximum entropy method does require considerable computing resources, processing times of several hours being needed with current clinical data processing systems. The use of an array processor will reduce this time.

8.3.3   Enhancing filters

Giver prior knowledge of the structures of interest, or the way in which they are masked by other image detail, it may be possible to emphasise particular image features so as to enhance the perceptibility of these structures. In contrast to the two previous categories of filter which were concerned mainly with rectifying deficiencies in the imaging process, namely noise and poor spatial resolution, the enhancing filter may actually distort the overall image appearance to achieve the desired result.

The simple differentiating filter (Fig. 8.17) emphasises the higher frequencies at the expense of low ones, so sharpening edges and assisting in the differentiation of lesions from adjacent anatomical structures. A similar result has been achieved by "unsharp masking", a process in which an image smoothed once with a nine-point filter (Section 8.3.1) has subtracted from it the same image processed several times with the same nine-point filter. This is an extremely simple, yet flexible, form of an enhancing filter.

Neill and Hutchinson (1971) have proposed a filter which specifically looks for the localised convexities (or concavities) in an image which may represent a lesion.

8.3.4   Usefulness of filters

Despite the variety of filters available, there has been a marked reluctance to apply them in clinical practice, apart from the simple nine-point smoothing filter. Two factors may have contributed to this situation: first, the reticence of clinicians to use data which has been 'manipulated' and second, the impression frequently given that for a filter to be useful it must be of value in all circumstances.

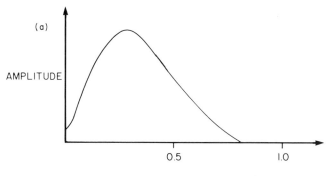

SPATIAL FREQUENCY, cm⁻¹

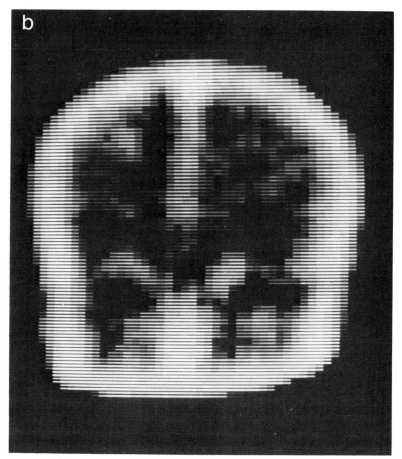

FIG. 8.17. (a) Differentiating filter and (b) brain image after processing with this filter.

Perhaps a more profitable approach would be to present the clinician with the original, unprocessed image together with versions of the same image processed using a selection of filters. The filters used on the supplementary images would have been chosen to deal with problems of interpretation peculiar to the particular clinical study. The observer's confidence in possible abnormal features seen on the processed images could then be tested against the unprocessed image.

In an intercomparison of filtering techniques using a set of brain images to which computer simulated abnormalities had been added (Houston *et al.*, 1979), observers were presented with images processed with a differentiating filter or with a convexity-seeking filter as well as with the original image. The differentiating filter was chosen to aid detection of lesions situated close to the edge of normal anatomical structures, while it was hoped that the convexity filter would improve the detection of those lesions in the middle of the almost uniform low uptake over the cerebral hemispheres. In comparison with other standard filtering techniques considered in the study it performed well. With the increasing power of nuclear medicine computer systems, such an approach should be simple to implement and incorporate into routine clinical work without unduly extending the time needed to interpret an image.

8.4 Concluding remarks

The ability to quantify data is undoubtedly a very useful tool in clinical radionuclide imaging. While it is difficult to measure the absolute amount of activity in an organ, relative changes can be accurately and easily measured. The production of time–activity curves is, perhaps, the principal use of the data-processing system.

Two areas of development have deen discussed, namely, the deconvolution of curves to give more precise data about organ handling of the radiopharmaceutical and functional images. In practice, the efficacy of both techniques is dependent upon the amount of noise in the image. Unfortunately, in some circumstances where deconvolution would be very helpful, such as when the injection has been partially extravasated or when the kidneys are functioning very poorly, the photon density is likely to prove too low for deconvolution to be reliable.

Functional imaging is a potentially useful method of image presentation, but has not gained wide acceptance. Its effectiveness is often limited by lack of understanding of the kinetics of the radiopharmaceutical and hence the difficulty in selecting suitable physiologically relevant indices.

Much work has been carried out in the area of image filtering. While there is no doubt that for certain specific tasks, such as edge detection, it can be of great value, its general application for enhancing the detectability of lesions in an image is more contentious. It is unrealistic to look for a filter which would enable previously undetectable lesions to be seen if only because it is doubtful whether, in the absence of other clinical evidence, the results would be accepted. Filters are best used to increase confidence in the presence of a lesion which is only visualised poorly on the unprocessed image.

The intrinsically poor quality of radionuclide images offers a challenge to data processing techniques. It is perhaps not unduly critical to say that this challenge has not yet been met fully. To a certain extent the problems lie in the relatively low computing power available in the average clinical data processing system, and it is to be hoped that with rapid development of technology, further progress will be made.

References

Alderson, P. O., Douglass, K. H., Mendenhall, K. G., Gundiana, V. A., Watson, D. C., Links, J. M. and Wagner, H. N. (1979). Deconvolution analysis in radionuclide quantitation of left to right cardiac shunts. *J. Nucl. Med.* **20**, 502–506.

Andrews, H. C. (1972). "Introduction to Mathematical Techniques in Pattern Recognition", pp. 15–32, John Wiley, New York.

Barber, D. C. (1976). Digital computer processing of brain scans using principal components. *Phys. Med. Biol.* **21**, 792–803.

Barber, D. C. (1980). The use of principal components in the quantitative analysis of gamma-camera dynamic studies. *Phys. Med. Biol.* **25**, 283–292.

Barber, D. C. and Nijran, K. S. (1981). Factor analysis of rose bengal liver function studies. *In* "Medical Image Processing", (M. L. Goris, ed.) pp. 32–55, Stanford University Press, Stanford, California.

Barber, D. C., Duthie, H. L., Howlett, P. J. and Ward, A. S. (1974). Principal components. A new approach to the analysis of gastric emptying. *In* "Dynamic Studies with Radioisotopes in Medicine" Vol. 1, pp. 185–195, IAEA, Vienna.

Bašić, M., Sharp, P. F. and Dendy, P. P. (1983). A functional imaging routine for cholescintigraphy. *Phys. Med. Biol.* **28**, 731–738.

Bazin, J. P., Di Paola, R., Gibaud, B., Rougier, P. and Tubiana, M. (1980). Factor analysis of dynamic scintigraphic data as a modelling method. An application to the detection of metastases. *In* "Information Processing in Medical Imaging" (R. Di Paola and E. Kahn, eds.), pp. 345–366, INSERM, Paris.

Blackman, R. B. and Tukey, J. W. (1958). "The Measurement of Power Spectra". Dover, New York.

Bossuyt, A., Deconinck, F., Lepoudre, R. and Jonckheer, M. (1980). The temporal Fourier transform applied to functional isotopic imaging. *In* "Information Processing in Medical Imaging" (R. Di Paola and E. Kahn, eds.), pp. 397–408, INSERM, Paris.

Britton, K. E., Granowska, M. and Nimmon, C. E. (1980). Total and regional cerebral blood flow. *In* "Medical Radionuclide Imaging", Vol. 1, pp. 315–322, IAEA, Vienna.

Chang, W., Henkin, R. E., Hale, D. J. and Hall, D. (1980). Methods for detection of left ventricular edges. *Semin. Nucl. Med.* **10**, 39–52.

Clarke, D. N., Sharp, P. F., Brunt, P. W., Mowat, N. A. G., Dascombe, G. and Smith, F. W. (1982). Hepatobiliary imaging using 99m-Tc pyridoxylidene glutamate in the diagnosis of obstructive jaundice. *Eur. J. Nucl. Med.* **7**, 370–375.

Diffey, B. L. and Corfield, J. R. (1976). Data bounding techniques in discrete deconvolution. *Med. Biol. Eng.* **14**, 478.

Diffey, B. L., Hall, F. M. and Corfield, J. R. (1976). The 99m-Tc DTPA dynamic renal scan with deconvolution analysis. *J. Nucl. Med.* **17**, 352–355.

Erickson, J. J. and Rollo, F. D. (1983). "Digital Nuclear Medicine". J. B. Lippincott, Philadelphia, Pennsylvania.

Ferrant, A. and Cauwe, F. (1979). Quantitative organ uptake measurement with a gamma-camera. *Eur. J. Nucl. Med.* **4**, 223–229.

Fleming, J. S. (1979). A technique for the absolute measurement of activity using a gamma-camera and computer. *Phys. Med. Biol.* **24**, 176–180.

Fleming, J. S. and Kenny, R. W. (1977). A comparison of techniques for the filtering of noise in the renogram. *Phys. Med. Biol.* **22**, 359–364.

Frieden, B. R. (1972). Restoring with maximum likelihood and maximum entropy. *J. Opt. Soc. Am.* **62**, 511–518.

Goris, M. L., Daspit, S. G., McLaughlin, P. and Kross, J. P. (1976). Interpolative background subtraction. *J. Nucl. Med.* **17**, 744–747.

Gull, S. F. and Daniell, G. J. (1978). Image reconstruction from incomplete and noisy data. *Nature (London)* **272**, 686–690.

Ham, J. R., Dobbelier, A., Viart, P., Piepsz, A. and Lenaers, A. (1981). Radionuclide quantitation of left to right cardiac shunts using deconvolution analysis. *J. Nucl. Med.* **22**, 688–692.

Houston, A. S. and MacLeod, M. A. (1980). Processing of liver dynamic studies with technetium-labelled sulphur colloid. *Br. J. Radiol.* **53**, 87–92.

Houston, A. S., Sharp, P. F., Tofts, P. S. and Diffey, B. L. (1979). A multicentre comparison of computer assisted image processing and display methods in scintigraphy. *Phys. Med. Biol.* **24**, 547–558.

Houston, A. S., Elliott, A. T. and Stone, D. L. (1982). Factorial phase imaging: a new concept in the analysis of first-pass cardiac studies. *Phys. Med. Biol.* **27**, 1269–1277.

Kemp, M. C. (1981). Maximum entropy reconstructions in emission tomography. *In* "Medical Radionuclide Imaging", Vol. 1, pp. 313–323, IAEA, Vienna.

Kenny, R. W., Ackery, D. M., Fleming, J. S., Goddard, B. A. and Grant, R. W. (1975). Deconvolution analysis of the scintillation camera renogram. *Br. J. Radiol.* **48**, 481–486.

King, M. A., Doherty, P. W., Rosenberg, R. J. and Cool, S. L. (1983). Array processors: an introduction to their architecture, software and applications in nuclear medicine. *J. Nucl. Med.* **24**, 1072–1079.

Metz, C. E. (1969). A mathematical investigation of radioisotope scan image processing. Ph.D. Thesis, University of Pennsylvania. University Microfilms, Ann Arbor, Michigan, Publication 70-16-186.

Miller, T. R. and Sampathkumaran, K. S. (1982). Digital filtering in nuclear medicine. *J. Nucl. Med.* **23**, 693–701.

Neill, G. D. S. and Hutchinson, F. (1971). Computer detection and display of focal lesions on scintigrams. *Br. J. Radiol.* **44**, 962–969.

Oppenheim, B. E. and Appledorn, C. R. (1980). Functional renal imaging using factor analysis. *In* Information Processing in Medical Imaging" (R. Di Paola and E. Kahn, eds.,) pp. 321–334, INSERM, Paris.

Piepsz, A., Ham, H. R., Erbsmann, F., Hall, M., Diffey, B. L., Coggin, M. J., Hall, F. M., Lumbroso, J., Di Paola, R., Bazin, J. P., Di Paola, M. and Fries, D. (1982). A cooperative study on the clinical value of dynamic renal scanning with deconvolution analysis. *Br. J. Radiol.* **55,** 419–433.

Pitt, W. R. and Sharp, P. F. (1981). Reproducibility of gamma-camera data. *Phys. Med. Biol.* **26,** 693–701.

Reeve, J. and Crawley, J. C. W. (1974). Quantitative radioisotope renography: the derivation of physiological data by deconvolution analysis using a single injection technique. *Clin. Sci. Mol. Med.* **47,** 317–330.

Ronai, P. M., Baker, R. J., Bellen, J. C., Collins, P., Anderson, J. and Lander, H. (1975). Technetium-99m-pyridoxylidene glutamate: a new hepato-biliary radiopharmaceutical. II Clinical aspects. *J. Nucl. Med.* **16,** 728–737.

Rosenfeld, A. and Kak, A. C. (1976). "Digital Picture Processing", Vol. 2, Chap. 10, Academic Press, New York.

Schmidlin, P. (1979). Quantitative evaluation and imaging of functions using pattern recognition methods. *Phys. Med. Biol.* **24,** 385–395.

Sorenson, J. A. (1974). Quantitative measurement of radioactivity *in-vivo* by whole body counting. *In* "Instrumentation in Nuclear Medicine" (G. J. Hine and J. A. Sorenson, eds.), Chap. 9. Academic Press, New York.

Tanaka, E. and Iinuma, T. A. (1970). Approaches to optimal data processing in radioisotope imaging. *Phys. Med. Biol.* **15,** 683–694.

Todd-Pokropek, A. E. (1980). Image processing in nuclear medicine. *IEEE Trans. Nucl. Sci.* **NS-27,** 1080–1094.

Zierler, K. L. (1965). Equations for measuring blood flow by external monitoring of radioisotopes. *Circ. Res.* **16,** 309–321.

Chapter 9

Evaluation of the Clinical Effectiveness of *in vivo* Imaging

9.1 Introduction

By concentrating on the physics of the imaging process, it is easy to overlook the most important aspect of the subject, namely that *in vivo* imaging is not an end in itself but only a means to an end. The reason why scanners and cameras are built, and why money is invested to improve them, is to provide a service to medicine, and that service will be judged almost entirely by the accuracy of the diagnostic information it produces. Therefore, it is important to include a chapter in which some of the problems that arise when attempts are made to evaluate either new equipment or a new test are discussed in the clinical context.

Critical objective evaluation of each diagnostic test is important for three reasons. First it may be used to assess diagnostic reliability. For example, we know that a radionuclide examination for bone disease is very sensitive and very accurate, whereas that for pancreatic disease is not very reliable. However, unless image interpretation can be more objective, clinical colleagues do not know how much credence or "weight" to give a report, especially if it partially contradicts the results of another examination. Second, objective information allows areas of weakness to be more critically analysed and provides a better basis for comparison between different centres practising nuclear medicine. Finally, as Lusted (1977) has so clearly stated, medical ethics is not independent of economics. Although medical decision analysis studies will continue to be directed towards optimising the quantity of medical information, this will have to be done within a sound economic framework.

Critical evaluation may be applied to all types of clinical, laboratory, radiological and radionuclide investigations. The information would be useful in most situations and is of special importance when the outcome of the test can have a radical effect on the management or wellbeing of patients. In spite of this, only relatively few tests have been assessed in any quantitative manner. In a review of the rationale for the use of bone scans in malignant disease, McNeil (1978) emphasised that we know less about the response of cancer patients to treatment than we might because the extent and location of primary and recurrent disease have not been documented in detail. She commented that, although a literature search provided several hundred references on bone scanning in malignant disease, fewer than 20 gave the kind of information required for rational decision making. She concluded that systematic evaluation studies on bone scanning in a variety of malignant processes were urgently required.

The problem is further complicated by publications in which claims are made that cannot be substantiated. For example, in a comparison of emission computed tomography versus conventional scintigraphy for lung disease, Le Jeune *et al.* (1982) conceded that their series comprised too few patients for any firm conclusions as to the superiority of tomography over traditional scanning techniques or vice versa. Furthermore, they presented no independent evidence on the condition of the lungs of patients who had been studied. Nevertheless, the authors concluded: "There is no doubt however, that tomography gave more precise information about the site and extent of lung defects"!

Some reasons for the reluctance to undertake quantitative evaluation studies will now be considered, with particular reference to *in vivo* imaging.

9.2 Evaluations dependent primarily on binary decisions

In the simplest approach to quantitative evaluation, an attempt is made to ask and answer two questions: (i) Is the test result normal or abnormal? (ii) Is the case a true normal or true abnormal?

If simple "yes" or "no" answers can be given to each question, several forms of data analysis, all using non-parametric statistics, may be available. A method using a 2×2 decision matrix is probably the simplest (Table 9.1) and, with certain qualifications, the results of *in vivo* imaging studies can sometimes be simplified in this way. The data shown in Table 9.2 are derived from a prospective trial to study the contribution of a tomographic

TABLE 9.1. A general 2 × 2 decision matrix that may be used when there are only four possible outcomes to an investigation.

	Abnormal results	Normal results	Total
True abnormals	a	b	$a+b$
True normals	c	d	$c+d$
Totals	$a+c$	$b+d$	$a+b+c+d$

TABLE 9.2. Detection of tumours by radionuclide brain scanning with the aid of a tomographic view.

	Abnormal scan	Normal scan	Total
True abnormals	44	6	50
True normals	5	367	372
Total	49	373	422

section view to lesion detection by radionuclide brain scanning (Carril et al., 1979).

The test may then be described in several ways. First we may ask the very simple question, what is the overall, diagnostic accuracy or how many reports were correct? The answer is $(a+d)/(a+b+c+d) = (44+367)/(49+373)$ or 97.4%. However, in general, correct identification of abnormal cases is more important than correct identification of normal cases. Thus, "sensitivity", the ratio (abnormals detected)/(total abnormals), is more often quoted and in this example is $a/(a+b) = 44/50 = 88.0\%$. Occasionally, if the test is complementary to another examination, accurate identification of normal cases may be more important. The "specificity" is defined as the ratio of normals correctly identified to total normals, and in this example is $d/(c+d) = 367/372 = 98.8\%$. Finally, it is sometimes important to know the predictive value of a positive test. This is the ratio of abnormals correctly identified to total abnormal reports or here $a/(a+c) = 89.8\%$

Thus, we see that even in this very simple example, there is no such thing as the "accuracy" of an examination and the concept is only meaningful in the context of the value of the clinical information to be obtained or the cost or an incorrect diagnosis.

An additional complication arises if, in addition to classifying images as normal or abnormal, a "doubtful" category is permitted. Maublant et al. (1982) adopted this approach when comparing conventional scintigraphy and emission tomography with 201-Tl for the detection of myocardial infarction. Since there were two observers, further disagreement and hence uncertainty also arose from this source. For the purpose of calculating sensitivity, doubtful cases were included with the normals, but an alternative approach would be to quote a range of sensitivities, obtained by first assuming all the doubtful cases were incorrect (most pessimistic estimate) and then assuming they were all correct (most optimistic estimate). This type of approach was adopted by Ell and co-workers when comparing the accuracies of different imaging techniques used to assess the condition of the liver (Ell *et al.*, 1981).

Prevalence has an important effect on the predictive value of a test. For example, when sensitivity and specificity are both 95%, the predictive value of a positive test varies from 2% when the prevalence is only 0.1% to 95% when the prevalence is 50% (Lusted, 1978).

To accommodate possible variations in prevalence of the disease, some groups have applied Bayes Theorem to calculate the posterior probability of a given condition, given the test results and assuming different *a priori* probabilities. For a full account of this approach, the reader is referred to Shea (1978). Here we give only the principal features.

If the prior probability of disease or prevalence is $P(D_+)$, then the posterior probability of disease when the test result is abnormal is given by

$$P(D_+|T_+) = \frac{[a/(a+b)]P(D_+)}{[a/(a+b)]P(D_+) + [c/(c+d)]P(D_-)}$$

where $\qquad P(D_-) = [1 - P(D_+)]$

Similarly the posterior probability of disease when the test result is normal is given by

$$P(D_+|T_-) = \frac{[b/(a+b)]P(D_+)}{[b/(a+b)]P(D_+) + [d/(c+d)]P(D_-)}$$

From these probabilities, it is possible to calculate a discriminant factor $F = P(D_+|T_+) - P(D_+|T_-)$ which is a numerical measure of the ability of the test to detect the presence of disease for a given prevalence.

Values of $P(D_+|T_+)$, $P(D_+|T_-)$ and F are then calculated for different assumed values of prevalence $P(D_+)$ and results such as those shown in Fig. 9.1 are obtained. These curves are taken from published work by Murray *et al.* (1981) to investigate the diagnostic value of stress 201-Tl scintigraphy for different prevalences of coronary heart disease.

The 45° lines in Figs. 9.1a and 9.1b would be obtained if the test contributed nothing since the posterior and prior probabilities are equal. Thus, the distance of the curve above the line in Fig. 9.1a and the distance of the curve below the line in Fig. 9.1b measures the power of the test. This

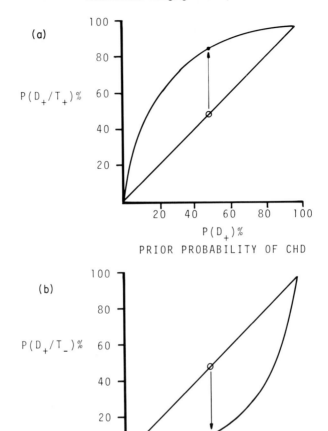

F$_{IG}$. 9.1. Use of Bayes Theorem to predict the influence of disease prevalence on the diagnostic value of a given test result. (a) The probability of having coronary heart disease (CHD) with a positive 201-Tl scintiscan $P(D_+|T_+)$, for CHD prevalences $P(D_+)$ ranging from 1 to 99%. At a prevalence of 50% (○), a positive test increased the probability of disease to 87% (●). (b) The probability of having CHD with a negative 201-Tl scintiscan, $P(D_+|T_-)$ for CHD prevalences ranging from 1 to 99%. At a prevalence of 50% (○) a negative test decreased the probability of disease to 10% (●). (c) Influence of prior probability of having CHD, $P(D_+)$, on the discriminant expression F. The discriminant value of 201-Tl scintigraphy falls sharply when the prior probability of CHD is below 30% or above 70%. [From Murray et al. (1981).]

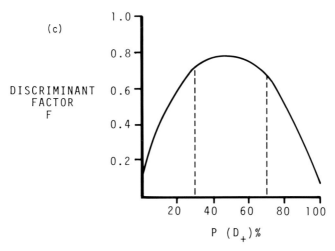

(c)

FIG. 9.1. (*Continued*)

work showed that the discriminant value of the test was highest when the prior probability of coronary heart disease was between 30% and 70% but was very low if the prevalance of disease was either very high or very low (Fig. 9.1c).

Strauss *et al.* (1982) used a similar approach to compare 99m-Tc sulphur colloid single-photon emission computed tomography (SPECT) with conventional scintigraphy for the identification and assessment of liver metastases. Results showed that SPECT had greater sensitivity, specificity and accuracy than conventional scans and was superior at all disease prevalences. However, a weakness of this study was the need to assume that results obtained by transmission computed tomography at the same time were unequivocally correct and to compare other techniques on this basis.

9.3 Evaluations based on ROC analysis

Thus far it has been assumed that only two results of the diagnostic examination are possible and that a clear boundary exists between them. In practice, the majority of tests give a continuous scale of abnormality and an arbitrary distinction must be made between normals and abnormals. None of the methods discussed so far allows for the possibility that the working point at which this distinction is made may vary. Any variation in this working point is essentially a trade-off between high sensitivity and high specificity. If it is made consciously, it must be in terms of the relative cost, both to the patient and to the service, of false positive and false negative decisions. Sometimes the variation may occur unconsciously, and this is most undesirable.

Account may be taken of such variations by using receiver operating characteristic analysis (ROC) and rating curves. These ideas were introduced in Chapter 7 in the context of perception studies on inanimate test objects. By awarding the set of scans obtained for each patient by *in vivo* imaging an abnormality rating from 0 to 5, this approach can be extended to clinical data. An example from our own work is shown in Table 9.3 and Fig. 9.2.

However, a number of additional problems must now be considered. First, the evaluation must be carried out within the reference frame of the normal routine work of the unit. Results obtained by a highly skilled operator working in a research environment are likely to overestimate quite markedly the diagnostic value of a new or modified procedure. Therefore, protocols must ensure that each set of images is given the same amount of attention when reported, neither more nor less than it would receive in normal practice. This precaution should also ensure automatically that a typical cross-section of normal images and abnormal images from different disease categories is sampled. We have already noted how prevalence affects the predictive value of a positive test, so prevalence must not be distorted by the selection of cases which seem particularly suitable for the study in question. In model experiments using ROC and rating curves, it is customary to attempt to use approximately equal

TABLE 9.3. Data collected using the Aberdeen section scanner with tomography for liver imaging.

True abnormals					
Abnormality rating	5	4	3	2	1	0
Number of cases	95	55	39	22	19	5
Cumulative total	95	150	189	211	230	235
Cumulative percentage	40	64	80	90	98	100
Normal deviate of cumulative percentage	-0.25	0.36	0.84	1.28	2.05	—

True normals					
Abnormality rating	5	4	3	2	1	0
Number of cases	7	10	17	15	50	39
Cumulative total	7	17	34	49	99	138
Cumulative percentage	5	12	25	36	72	100
Normal deviate of cumulative percentage	-1.65	-1.17	-0.67	-0.36	0.58	—

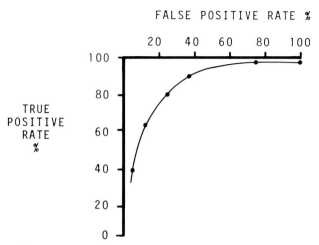

FIG. 9.2. ROC curve derived from the data in Table 9.3.

numbers of true positive and true negative cases (Metz, 1978). In clinical practice, because of the need to sample a typical cross section of the disease categories, it is rarely possible to do this. For example, in our prospective trial to study the value of transverse section imaging for lesion detection in the brain, there were 372 independently confirmed normal cases but only 140 independently confirmed abnormal cases (Carril *et al.*, 1979). This imbalance introduces considerable asymmetry in the x and y directions when error bars are put on the ROC curves.

The error bars shown in Fig. 9.3 represent the standard deviation of the variation that can be expected in any one plotted operating point, calculated according to the method of Green and Swets (1966). Although this is a useful exercise for visual interpretation, in the context of clinical evaluation it is suspect. For example, very frequently, as here, two diagnostic tests are being applied to the same patient population so the ROC curves are not generated from statistically independent data. Since binomial variance fails to take account of this, the significance or curve separation in such a situation may be underestimated. On the other hand neither does binomial variance account fully for biological or psychological variability of observers, or variability of the systems tested, all of which can be expected to increase the magnitude of the error bar. A further problem is that large numbers of cases are required to achieve statistical accuracy, yet for many types of investigation one wishes to analyse, the number of cases in any one centre is very small. Finally, since data along one line are cumulative, the points are not independent. In a review of the application of ROC curve analysis to clinical data, Turner (1978) suggested that no entirely satisfactory statistical method had yet been described.

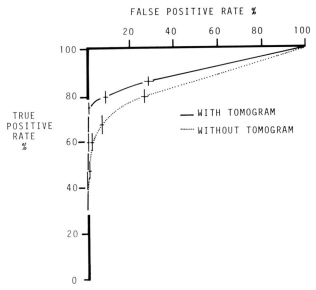

F<small>IG</small>. 9.3. ROC curves produced in a prospective trial to examine the effect of tomographic section images on diagnostic accuracy in radionuclide brain examinations. The curves suggest better results with the tomogram. The error bars give some indication of the accuracy of the data. [From Carril *et al.* (1979).]

In recent years considerable attention has been devoted to the assignment of a single index of diagnostic accuracy to the ROC curve, and the most comprehensive treatment is by Swets and Pickett (1982). The starting point for a mathematical approach has been an empirical assumption, but one that has nevertheless been validated in a large number of diverse applications. It is that the varying degrees of normality or abnormality seen in images can be represented by two separate Gaussian distributions, one for the diseased group and one for the non-diseased group.

Making this assumption, then if the data are plotted on binomial graph paper, or the normal deviates of the probability are scaled linearly, the result should be straight line. Figure 9.4 shows the data of Table 9.3 handled in this way. A straight line may be fitted by eye and it can be seen that the fit is quite good. Alternatively, the data may easily be fitted by statistical techniques that give the maximum likelihood of the slope and intercept of the line.

A number of measurements have been suggested for describing the curve but the proportion of the ROC space lying below the graph A_z is the most popular and is the easiest to appreciate visually. Reference to Fig. 8.11 shows that A_z varies from 0.5, when the ROC curve is based on guess-work, to 1.0, when the decision process is totally accurate.

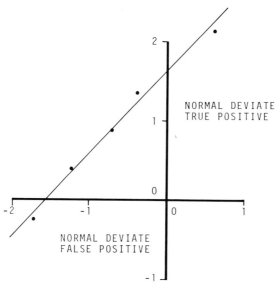

FIG. 9.4. Plot obtained when the normal deviates of the percentage points in FIG. 9.2 are displayed on a linear–linear scale.

One simple way to estimate A_z is to join pairs of points in Fig. 9.2 and use the trapezoidal rule. This avoids assumptions concerning the form of the probability distribution, but if the points are not well spread across the ROC curve, it under-estimates the value A_z. Preferable methods are to use the slope and intercept of the original data when plotted on binormal graph paper or to use a maximum likelihood estimation programme. In Swets and Pickett (1982) a slightly modified version of a maximum likelihood method first published by Dorfman and Alf (1969) is given. The value of A_z calculated in this way for the data shown in Table 9.3 and Fig. 9.4 was 86%.

A number of papers have appeared that address some of the outstanding problems associated with the use of ROC curves. Hanley and McNeil (1982) have investigated the meaning and use of the index A_z to describe an ROC curve. They were able to show that the relationship of A_z to the Wilcoxon statistic could be used to describe its statistical properties such as standard error, and the sample sizes required to measure the area with a pre-specified degree of precision.

Both this work and the computer programme of Dorfman and Alf, which requires certain minimal frequencies in each response category, suggest that quite large numbers of cases will be required. Therefore Hermann *et al.* (1982) have examined the performance characteristics of multi-reader groups by asking members of the College of American Pathologists Phantom-Imaging Series to report independently on a set of test images. At present the study has been confined to a laboratory exercise with care being taken to avoid introducing clinical factors. Nevertheless, the survey did demonstrate the feasibility of deriving indices of group performance in visual detection tasks using peer group survey techniques that provide access to relatively large numbers of suitable observers.

Hanley and McNeil (1983) have also reported a method for comparing A_z values when the data for the two ROC curves are derived from the same patients. This method takes into account the correlation between the areas that is induced by the paired nature of the data. This approach, which is analogous to the use of a paired t-test, can reduce the standard error on the observed differences in areas, thereby giving a considerable increase in the statistical sensitivity of the comparison. When studies involve multiple readers, this method also provides a measure of this component of the sampling variation that is otherwise difficult to obtain.

Mould (1979) has called for even greater precision than the six point abnormality rating scale described here and has suggested that probability statements should be attached to scan reports. Such statements can be regarded as giving the risk of making a wrong decision. If q_n is the probability of the organ being normal, then $q_a = (1 - q_n)$ is the probability that the organ is abnormal. If patient records including q_n or q_a values from organ image reports are stored on the computer, they can be updated with autopsy or operative findings and an assessment can be made of how often normality is proved for various q_n values or abnormality proven for various q_a values.

Whilst it is important to focus attention on this point, it may be unrealistic to expect very great precision in clinical interpretation, since not only physical features of the scan appearance but also clinical factors are relevant. The latter can rarely be quantified because of a lack of internal standards but nevertheless must contribute to the final abnormality rating. For example, it is a matter of common experience that liver images become progressively more irregular with increasing average age of patients, but should this be recorded as an abnormality, since in the absence of any other liver pathology it is unlikely to affect the patient's health or to be detected by any other diagnostic test?

Abnormality ratings of 0, 1, 2, 3, 4, 5, correspond to rounded probability statements of 0%, 20%, 40%, ... etc., and we have shown that, even using this relatively coarse scale, it is difficult to assess consistently the degree of abnormality. When the same set of scans, some of which had been selected because of features that might make interpretation difficult, were shown to different teams of observers, there was a difference in the abnormality rating awarded in half of the cases (Dendy *et et al.*, 1977). This suggested that greater precision may not be justified and might give a misleading impression of the reliability of scan interpretation.

9.4 Trial design

Retrospective trials may be of value as feasibility studies but should be followed by prospective trials. When Sostre *et al.* (1978) evaluated retrospectively gamma-camera images obtained with a pinhole camera against rectilinear scans for the identification of thyroid abnormalities, clinically established "true" diagnoses were determined in advance by two independent observers using all available information including biochemical and immunological tests, surgery where appropriate, and scintigraphy. All cases were allocated to one of five disease categories: normal, single cold nodule, single hot nodule, multinodular and heterogeneous. Then four different observers re-evaluated and categorised the scan data alone. By using an expanded decision matrix and multivariate information analysis, it was possible to study not only the overall accuracy of the two imaging methods, but also the observers' ability to identify specific disease patterns. The authors were able to calculate five parameters—sensitivity, specificity, signal detection accuracy or overall percentage accuracy, signal identification accuracy and the information transmitted—all of which indicated that the pinhole camera was superior to rectilinear scanning for thyroid 99m-Tc imaging with pertechnetate. This paper made an important contribution to methods of analysing diagnostic data. However, the retrospective nature of the study was a limitation because it meant that clinical details which would normally be available had to be withheld from the four observers engaged in the study. It has been shown that withholding such details causes artefacts, particularly in deciding the disease category, because even a brief clinical history makes an important contribution towards this decision (Carril *et al.*, 1979).

In evaluating any diagnostic information, the problem of independent, unequivocal identification of true normal and true abnormal cases is well recognised. Furthermore, the reliability with which this can be done may vary for different parts of the body. For example, the presence of a tumour or metastasis in the brain will quickly be confirmed by other symptomatic changes. For the liver, the situation is much more complex. A laparotomy will certainly not be performed unless there are other good reasons to do so, and a needle biopsy, even if taken, may miss the tumour. On the other hand, with good chemotherapy the patient may survive a long time even if liver metastases are present. Hence the exact state of the liver at the time of radionuclide examination may never be known.

Because the exact clinical condition of the patient often cannot be determined by independent methods, many papers stop short of a full evaluation of a new test. For example, Hauser and Gottschalk (1978) investigated the contribution of tomographic section views for imaging gallium distributions within the patient, especially in the abdomen and thorax. They found that tomographic scanner views were preferred to gamma camera views for 49% of cases, camera views were preferred for 12%, and 39% were equivalent. Whilst these conclusions are useful, it is important to emphasise that they represent preferences for interpretation by experienced nuclear medicine physicians. This falls some way short of the conclusion that conventional plus tomographic images are more accurate than conventional views alone for this particular study.

In recent work on the role of tomographic scintigraphy for identification of liver disease, Reid *et al.* (1983) attempted to allow for variation in the reliability of independent data on the condition of the liver by introducing a diagnostic rating. As shown in Table 9.4, on this rating scale reliable, independent evidence gives either a very high or a very low rating. Less reliable evidence results in an intermediate rating.

Receiver operating characteristic curves could than be constructed using different working points on the diagnostic classification rating scale to distinguish between true normal and true abnormal livers. Alternatively, the analysis could be restricted to cases where the diagnostic rating was high. As shown in Fig. 9.5, well-confirmed abnormal cases were identified with a higher degree of confidence when observers had the benefit of the tomographic image.

TABLE 9.4. A variable rating for independent evidence on the liver condition.[a]

Diagnostic rating	Direct test results[b]	Indirect test results
0	negative	negative
1	negative	positive/conflicting
2	none	more than one negative
3	none	one/majority negative
4	none	conflicting equally
5	none	one/majority positive
6	none	more than one positive
7	positive	negative/conflicting
8	positive	positive

[a] From Reid *et al.* (1983).
[b] Biopsy post-mortem and laparotomy are considered direct results.

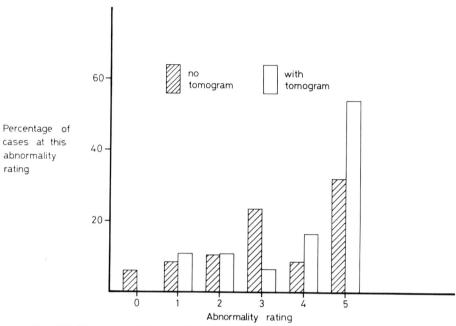

Fig. 9.5. Histograms of abnormality ratings allocated to liver scans, either with or without tomograms when only followed up cases with a confirmed diagnostic rating of 6 or higher (see Table 9.4) were considered. [From Reid *et al.* (1983).]

A well-designed clinical trial should also provide indications for further improvement. For example, the results of our first trial using a section scanner to assess the contribution of a tomographic image to liver scintigraphy suggested that sensitivity was high, 92% correct identification of focal disease with the tomogram, but specificity was disappointing with only about 75% correct identification of livers considered normal by other examinations. Thus, we knew the major weakness in our reporting, and when the second trial was initiated using a rotating gamma camera, an effort was made not to over-report the tomographic images. The results of the second trial showed little change in sensitivity, either for all cases or for the sub-groups of focal and diffuse disease. However, there was considerable improvement in the correct identification of true normals, particularly with the tomogram. This may have resulted from

(i)   the use of a high resolution gamma camera to produce conventional images

(ii)   availability of multiple section images from gamma camera tomography

TABLE 9.5. Values of A_z derived from ROC curves for two prospective trials to evaluate the contribution to diagnostic accuracy of section views through the liver.

	A_z without tomogram	A_z with tomogram
Aberdeen section scanner	86%	86%
Rotating gamma camera	89%	95%

(iii)   a conscious change in decision criteria during reporting

(iv)   a combination of all three.

As shown in Table 9.5, progress could be assessed in numerical terms because the trials had been designed and carried through in a consistent manner. Using the concept of A_z, it was possible to show that diagnostic accuracy was improved by changing from the scanner to the camera and was best when the camera was used with tomography. For further details see Dendy and Gemmell (1983).

9.5   Comparison of imaging procedures

With reference to *in vivo* imaging, it is important to distinguish two types of clinical evaluation. The first is an internal comparison between two *in vivo* imaging devices, for example a scanner and a camera or two cameras, which both use the single-photon emission principle. The second is an external comparison where radionuclide imaging is compared with some competing or complementary investigation such as ultrasonic examination or biochemical tests. Each approach is subject to other constraints in addition to those already discussed. For example, a dynamic study cannot be repeated on the same patient for the purpose of gamma-camera evaluation since it is ethically inadmissible to administer the second injection because of the unnecessary additional radiation exposure.

A number of papers have been published in which scintigraphy has been compared with other diagnostic imaging techniques. Snow *et al.* (1979) compared scintigraphy, ultrasound and computed tomography for the evaluation of hepatic neoplasms. Either positive histology or unequivocal sub-selective angiographic findings, or sometimes both, within 1 month of the scans was taken as positive proof of disease. Their results showed computed tomography to be more sensitive, more specific and more accurate than scintigraphy, which in turn was better than ultrasound. When diagnosis was based on two positive tests, computed tomography and scintigraphy combined were most successful. However, the fact that on numerous occasions tumour was correctly identified by two tests but missed by the third highlights the problems that arise when test results disagree.

Two recent papers (Cimitan *et al.*, 1983; Buell *et al.*, 1983) which have compared scintigraphy with ultrasound for the identification of liver disease should be mentioned. Both groups claimed that the combined use of the two techniques produced the best accuracy but did not explain how the data were combined in cases where there was disagreement. It is difficult to understand how sensitivity could be improved without loss of specificity or vice versa.

This view is in accord with the findings of McNeil *et al.* (1981) who compared computed tomography, ultrasound and gallium citrate imaging in patients with fever. Use of ROC curves showed no significant difference in the ability of the three modalities to differentiate focal from non-focal sources of sepsis. If a positive result was scored when either of the two examinations was abnormal, sensitivity increased from 60% to nearly 90%, but the false positive rate increased from 15% to 25%.

Particular care must be exercised when attempting to introduce a completely new mode of diagnostic investigation since premature introduction of an improperly evaluated technique could, in the worst instance, be a disaster since it might result in a proven technique being replaced by an inferior one. Moskowitz *et al.* (1983) have identified three distinct developmental stages through which any new technique must pass:

(i)   clinical feasibility which will determine if the new method has any potential,

(ii)   clinical suitability which will decide if the technology and diagnostic criteria are capable of being transferred to other institutions and other interpreters,

(iii)   verification of screening capability in which the power of the new method to complement or replace existing techniques will be assessed.

Although this article was written within the framework of new imaging procedures for breast cancer, where radionuclide imaging has no foreseeable role, many of the points are relevant to the introduction of any new diagnostic technique for a study of any part of the body. The complete process will be complex and lengthy, and as a salutary reminder that medicine is cost-limited, Moskowitz *et al.* (1983) devoted a lengthy paragraph to consideration of how the evaluation would be funded and (in America) what proportion of the cost the patient would be expected to pay.

For external comparisons, two further points must be emphasised. First, one must compare equivalent technologies. It is meaningless to compare the results obtained using a 1975 model ultrasonic scanner with those obtained using a 1983 model gamma camera or vice versa, because significant improvements will have been made to both devices during the intervening 8 years. The second point is that, as has already been noted, it is impossible to eliminate completely the subjective element from test reporting. Evaluation must therefore be designed so that the skill and experience of the reporting teams do not influence the final result. This is always difficult and sometimes impossible to achieve and there are no simple solutions. Nevertheless, the problem must be clearly recognised.

9.6 Concluding remarks

In conclusion, it is clear that until relatively recently little thought had been given to the question of critical clinical evaluation of diagnostic tests, especially *in vivo* radionuclide imaging investigations. However, designs for good prospective clinical trials are now being worked out, many of the problems have been identified, and it is possible to assess much more accurately the contribution of each diagnostic examination within the larger framework of patient health care.

References

Buell, U., Kessler, M., Kirsch, C. M. and Roedler, H. D. (1983). Letter re single photon emission computed tomography (SPECT) for assessment of hepatic lesions. Its role in the diagnostic work-up. *J. Nucl. Med.* **24**, 746.

Carril, J. M., MacDonald, A. F., Dendy, P. P., Keyes, W. I., Undrill, P. E. and Mallard, J. R. (1979). Cranial scintigraphy: value of adding emission computed tomographic sections to conventional pertechnetate images (512 cases). *J. Nucl. Med.* **20**, 1117–1123.

Cimitan, M., Spaziante, R., Pasquotti, G., Bruno, A. and Zecchin, R. (1983). Ultrasonic and scintigraphic imaging for malignant liver tumours in heavy drinkers. *Eur. J. Nucl. Med.* **8**, 105–108.

Dendy, P. P. and Gemmell, H. G. (1983). An evaluation of the contribution of single photon emission computed tomography (SPECT) to radionuclide imaging of the liver. *Ann. Radiol.* **26**, 72–81.

Dendy, P. P., McNab, T. W., MacDonald, A. F., Keyes, W. I. and Undrill, P. E. (1977). An evaluation of transverse axial tomography of the brain. *Br. J. Radiol.* **50**, 555–561.

Dorfman, D. B. and Alf, E., Jr. (1969). Maximum likelihood estimation of parameters of signal detection theory and determination of confidence intervals. Rating method data. *J. Math. Psychol.* **6**, 487–496.

Ell, P. J., Khan, O., Jarritt, P. H. and Radia, R. G. (1981). The clinical role of single photon emission tomography. *In* "Medical Radionuclide Imaging 1980", Vol. 1, pp. 255–262. IAEA, Vienna.

Green, D. M. and Swets, J. A. (1966). "Signal Detection Theory and Psychophysics", p.401. John Wiley, New York.

Hanley, J. A. and McNeil, B. J. (1982). The meaning and use of the area under a receiver operating characteristic (ROC) curve. *Radiology* **143**, 29–36.

Hanley, J. A. and McNeil, B. J. (1983). A method of comparing the areas under Receiver Operating Characteristic Curves derived form the same cases. *Radiology* **148**, 839–843.

Hauser, M. F. and Gottschalk, A. (1978). A comparison of the Anger tomographic scanner and the 15 inch scintillation camera for gallium imaging. *J. Nucl. Med.* **19**, 1074–1077.

Hermann, G. A., Herrera, N. and Suguira, H. T. (1982). Comparison of interlaboratory survey data in terms of receiver operator characteristic indices. *J. Nucl. Med.* **23**, 525–531.

Le Jeune, J. J., Maublant, J., Lehallac, M. and Veyre, A. (1982). Emission computed tomography vs. perfusion scanning in lung disease. *Eur. J. Nucl. Med.* **7**, 171–173.

Lusted, L. B. (1977). An analysis of medical decision making. *In* "Medical Radionuclide Imaging" Vol. 1, p. 185. IAEA, Vienna.

Lusted, L. B. (1978). General problems in medical decision making with comments on ROC analysis. *Semin. Nucl. Med.* **8**, 299–306.

McNeil, B. J. (1978). Rationale for the use of bone scans in selected metastatic and primary bone tumours. *Semin. Nucl. Med.* **8**, 336–345.

McNeil, B. J., Sanders, R., Alderson, P. O., Hessel, S. J., Finberg, H. J., Siegelman, S. S., Adams, D. F. and Abrams, H. L. (1981). A prospective study of computed tomography, ultrasound and gallium imaging in patients with fever. *Radiology* **139**, 647–653.

Maublant, J., Cassagnes, J., LeJeune, J. J., Mestas, D., Veyre, A., Jallut, H. and Meyniel, G. (1982). A comparison between conventional scintigraphy and emission tomography with thallium 201 in the detection of myocardial infarction. *J. Nucl. Med.* **23**, 204–208.

Metz, C. E. (1978). Basic principles of ROC analysis. *Semin. Nucl. Med.* **8**, 283–298.

Moskowitz, M., Feig, S. A., Cole-Beuglet, C., Fox, S. H., Haberman, J. D., Libshitz, H. I. and Zermeno, A. (1983). Evaluation of new imaging procedures for breast cancer: proper processes. *Am. J. Radiol.* **140**, 591–594.

Mould, R. F. (1979). Nuclear imaging and probability levels. *J. Nucl. Med.* **20**, 364.

Murray, R. G., McKillop, J. H., Bessent, R. G., Hutton, I., Lorimer, A. R. and Lawrie, T. D. V. (1981). Bayseian Analysis of stress Thallium-201 scintigraphy. *Eur. J. Nucl. Med.* **6**, 201–204.

Reid, A., Dendy, P. P., Gemmell, H. G. and Smith, F. W. (1983). Value of tomographic section views in identifying liver abnormalities by scintigraphy. *Acta Radiol. Diagn.* **24**, 107–111.

Shea, G. (1978). An analysis of the Bayes Procedure for diagnosing multistage disease. *Comput. Biomed. Res.* **11**, 65–75.

Snow, J. H., Goldstein, H. M. and Wallace, S. (1979). Comparison of scintigraphy, sonography and computed tomography in the evaluation of hepatic neoplasms. AJR, *Am. J. Roentgenol.* **132**, 915–918.

Sostre, S., Ashare, A. B., Quinones, J. D., Schieve, J. E. and Milton-Zimmerman, D. O. (1978). Thyroid scintigraphy versus rectilinear scans. *Radiology* **129**, 759–762.

Stauss, L., Bostel, F., Clorius, J. H., Ratou, E., Wellman, H. and Georgi, P. (1982). Single photon emission computed tomography (SPECT) for assessment of hepatic lesions. *J. Nucl. Med.* **23**, 1059–1065.

Swets, J. A. and Pickett, R. M. (1982). "Evaluation of Diagnostic Systems: Methods From Signal Detection Theory". Academic Press, New York and London.

Turner, D. A. (1978). An intuitive approach to receiver operating characteristic curve analysis. *J. Nucl. Med* **19**, 213–220.

Chapter 10

The Future

In this book we have attempted to present an in-depth account, written primarily from the view-point of the physicist, of the current status of *in vivo* diagnostic imaging using small quantities of radioactive material. From modest beginnings, the subject has developed rapidly during the past 25 years in many parts of the world. In western countries, radionuclide diagnostic examinations are now carried out at the rate of approximately 0.5% of the adult population per annum.

An important factor in the growth of the subject was the introduction of 99m-Tc. No other radionuclide has such a favourable combination of good physical properties and availability, and it is unlikely that the present situation, whereby over 90% of all investigations use 99m-Tc as the radioactive label, will change radically. Nevertheless, the degree of specificity of many radiopharmaceuticals remains extremely poor with frequently no more than a few percent of the administered activity localising in the region of interest. Thus, there is an urgent need to develop new radiopharmaceuticals that will concentrate in the organ of interest and that can be administered at the highest possible activity consistent with acceptable radiation dose to the patient.

The non-physiological nature of technetium is always going to be a limitation and alternative radionuclides are being considered seriously. An example is 123-I which has excellent physical properties and may be firmly bound to a wide range of biologically important molecules, especially proteins. A good example of its application has been the preparation of 123-I *N*-isopropyl *p*-iodoamphetamine. This radiopharmaceutical is lipid soluble and has a high extraction fraction in the brain. Differentiation of the grey and white matter of the basal ganglion has been achieved using this agent; acute infarctions have been demonstrated; and perfusion abnormalities are well shown (Hill et al., 1982). This radiopharmaceutical clearly has considerable potential for assessing regional brain perfusion. Unfortunately, 123-I will always be expensive to produce, since no generator system is available.

An important recent development has been in radiolabelled monoclonal antibodies for tumour imaging. Many attempts have been made in the past to use labelled anti-tumour antibodies for imaging and therapy and useful results have been reported using 131-I-labelled antibodies against many cancer-associated proteins notably carcino-embryonic antigen, alpha feto protein and human chorionic gonadotrophin. The major difficulties of such work have been associated with antibody preparation and purification and generally rather poor anti-tumour specificity.

The introduction of hybridoma technology capable of producing mono-clonal antibodies with greatly enhanced specificity for tumour-distinct markers has provided a powerful stimulus to such work. Two examples will be mentioned from a number of reports that have appeared in the literature. Larson et al. (1983) raised monoclonal antibodies against the human melanoma-associated antigen p.97 which is situated on the outer surface of the plasma membrane and is accessible to antigen. Six patients with malignant melanoma were treated, all had positive scans and, overall, 22 out of 25 lesions larger than 1.5 cm in diameter were visualised. Smedley et al. (1983) prepared rat monoclonal antibodies by immunising rats with human colorectal carcinoma cell membranes and fusing splenic lymphocytes with rat myeloma. A monoclonal which showed high binding activity on malignant compared to normal colon sections was selected and grown to large quantities in serum-free medium. The 131-I-labelled antibody was administered to 27 patients with colonic and other tumours and scintigrams were obtained at 48 h. Localised areas of uptake corresponding with known areas of disease were identified in 13 out of 16 cases of colorectal carcinoma and 3 out of 4 cases of breast carcinoma.

A major problem with labelled monoclonal antibodies is their relatively slow accumulation at the site of the tumour. Maximum levels are not reached until between 24 and 48 h after injection, so 99m-Tc labelling is unsuitable for such studies. In spite of the poor physical properties of its gamma radiations for imaging and the high beta dose to the patient, 131-I has been used for most work to date. Attempts are now being made to use 111-indium (111-In) which has excellent gamma rays for imaging at 172 and 247 keV but is technically much more difficult to attach firmly to the protein.

Even when imaging is delayed until 48 h, there are still high levels of free iodide and labelled protein in the blood pool. To correct for this, Smedley *et al.* (1983) injected 99m-Tc-labelled human serum albumen and 99m-Tc-labelled pertechnetate immediately prior to scanning and used computerised subtraction of the blood image pool. There is a need for further work to develop simple, more specific, background subtraction techniques, but the fact that background subtraction is necessary at all shows that most results obtained so far for tumour visualisation with monoclonal antibodies have been rather disappointing.

Another area of growing interest is the development of techniques for acid encapsulated in liposomes to image tumours in mice. Liposomes are small (approximately 1 μm), unilamellar lipid vesicles and many attempts have been made to employ them as carriers to protect and deliver therapeutic or diagnostic agents (Kaye, 1981). Profitt *et al.* (1983) have recently described an improved technique in which the liposomes were prepared from pure distearoyl phosphatidylcholine and cholesterol. They claim a maximum tumour-associated activity for EMT 6 tumours in BALB/c mice of 18% of the injected dose.

Many of the biologically important radionuclides are short half-life, positron emitting cyclotron products, notably 11-C, 13-N, 15-O and 18-F, and a wide range of radiopharmaceuticals have been prepared from one or other of these materials. A good example is 11-C deoxyglucose which has been used extensively for studies of cerebral glucose metabolism in man (Phelps, 1981).

Another area of growing interest is the development of techniques for the external detection and quantification of receptor sites in man. Receptors are substances on cell membranes or within cells that bind exogenous molecules or exogeneous drugs with high affinity. They may be detected by compounds such as 18-F haloperidol which is a ligand for the murine neuroleptic receptor. However, it is appropriate to insert a few words of caution here. The first step towards producing a new agent is to prepare a radioligand, labelled at sufficiently high specific activity, that will bind to the receptor satisfactorily and will provide a signal that can be measured externally. For the *in vitro* work, it is normal to prepare the tritiated analogue since tritium is easier to handle, has a longer half-life and is less expensive. However, care must be taken to ensure that the two analogues behave similarly *in vivo*. Zanzonico *et al.* (1983) have recently demonstrated that their preparations of 3-H haloperidol and 18-F haloperidol had completely different distributions and kinetic data *in vivo*. Re-examination of the results showed that after 1 h, very little of the tritium was still associated with the haloperidol and this was due to the tritium being exchanged off the ligand rather than the ligand being metabolised.

Only a few of the many new radiopharmaceuticals produced in recent years have been mentioned here. For example, there has been no mention of the wide range of labelled blood products. However, enough has been said to convince the reader that the intense activity in radiopharmaceutical research truly reflects the potential for progress in nuclear medicine in this area.

A second important factor in the growth of nuclear medicine was the introduction of a high-efficiency detector of gamma rays. This is the NaI(Tl) crystal scintillation detector which has very good properties for *in vivo* imaging. It is the basis of all currently available commercial imaging devices for routine work, now usually in the form of a gamma camera.

The performance of the gamma camera is, to a large extent, limited by the relatively few light photons produced from a photo-electric interaction of 99m-Tc gamma rays in a NaI(Tl) crystal. Most calculations suggest that technology is approaching the limit of intrinsic spatial resolution, with a practical achievable limit of about 3 mm FWHM at 140 keV.

The most promising alternative to the scintillation detector appears to be the solid-state detector. With such a detector, the greatly improved energy resolution resulting from the high yield of electron–hole pairs from each detected gamma ray permits more effective discrimination against scattered radiation. Introduction of large-field-of-view solid-state crystal detectors would clearly give a significant improvement but appears to be some way in the future. Rougeot *et al.* (1982) have recently examined progress in the use of solid state detectors in conjunction with image intensifiers, but even when such detectors are used in this way the field of view is rather small at present.

Whichever detector is chosen, imaging is still faced with two problems. The first is the need to produce an accurate representation of the three-dimensional distribution of radioactivity within the patient. This can never be achieved by a gamma camera operating in the conventional mode because the image is, to a certain extent, a superposition of activity in different planes. The problem can be largely overcome by single-photon emission computed tomography (SPECT) and much interest has been generated in this subject in recent years (see, e.g., Esser, 1983).

Several manufacturers have produced cameras that are capable of the necessary rotational movements; appropriate software is readily available; and some of the newer radiopharmaceuticals discussed earlier are particularly suitable for SPECT. To correct for attenuation in the patient, methods are available for simple, symmetrical, uniform problems such as the head, but for variable attenuation, iterative methods requiring expanded computing facilities are having to be introduced. It is still difficult, if not impossible, to extract quantitative data on radionuclide distributions from section images, and most methods contain a high degree of empiricism.

Most of the papers now being published seem to record some evidence of improved detection with SPECT. For example, Kirsch *et al.* (1983) showed higher sensitivity with SPECT than with computer-assisted conventional scintigraphy for detection of severe coronary heart disease with 201-thallium. However, a follow-up paper by Smalling (1983) raises recurring questions in connection with SPECT. Has the apparent "improvement" been achieved by depressing the sensitivity of the normal examination, and does the extra cost warrant the marginal improvement in the type of information obtained?

Closely related to SPECT is positron emission tomography (PET), and a recent potential improvement in PET is to make use of the spatial information that can be deduced from the time difference Δt between the arrival of the two 0.51-MeV gamma rays at the two detectors (Budinger, 1983). If Δx is the distance of the disintegrating source from the mid-point of the line joining the detectors, then $t = 2\Delta x/c$ where c is the speed of electromagnetic waves. It may be shown that, in theory, this information may be used to improve the signal to noise ratio by reducing the effective number of resolution elements and hence the noise associated with the Poisson statistics of a small number of counts per element. Furthermore, the use of time-of-flight information can greatly reduce the number of random coincidences recorded and can allow very high count rates to be handled. However, extremely fast electronics are required. If $\Delta x = 4.5$ cm then $\Delta t = 3 \times 10^{-10}$ s. In addition, if reasonably thick crystals, say of the order of 3 cm, are used to give adequate sensitivity, there is a significant timing error associated with variations in depth within the crystal at which the gamma ray is recorded. Although interesting work on PET is in progress at a number of research centres, it is unlikely to be introduced widely on a routine basis because of the high cost involved.

The second major problem for *in vivo* imaging is to find an efficient method of forming a gamma ray image on the detector, since the very low efficiency of collimators makes them the prime weakness in current imaging devices. The potential of two devices, the Compton-effect camera and coded aperture imaging, has already been discussed, but both have severe limitations and may not provide a widely applicable solution.

Quality control has become standard in many centres and a number of publications have appeared setting out recommended procedures for a gamma camera (WHO, 1982; Mould, 1983). The most important parameters of the system that should be measured are spatial resolution, both intrinsic and system, uniformity, count rate capability, sensitivity and energy resolution. It is also important to ensure adequate quality control of the camera–computer interface. Tests relating to the use of camera and computer for both static and dynamic imaging are required and if significant deviations from the performance at acceptance are found, it is important to find out if the problem is with the interface or with the camera.

Quality control in SPECT imposes more stringent requirements than conventional imaging, notably with respect to camera uniformity, and there are mechanical constraints associated with alignment and rotation. Any variation of camera response with angular position, for example as a result of stray magnetic fields, can cause serious problems (Jahangir *et al.*, 1983) and data correction procedures are still necessary to compensate for non-uniformity of detector response, attenuation, variations in point spread function of the camera, and the effects of scatter (Budinger, 1982).

Most work on quality control has been in terms of physical parameters of the systems, but there is now a need for work on quality control of gamma-camera *images* in which attempts are made to relate changes in physical parameters to perceived changes in images. On the basis of work with simple test objects, Kasal *et al.* (1983) have suggested that perceptible image deterioration will occur if the FWHM of the line spread function of the camera increases by 10% or more. This claim is now being investigated in studies on clinical images.

Considerable emphasis has been placed in this book on the importance of image display. The difficulty in making subjective measurements of the quality of clinical images means that there are still many unanswered questions: whether colour has any advantage over monochrome; whether analogue images are more effective than digitised images; whether filtering improves lesion detectability. It may be that no one display is best for all tasks; for example, in our experience, lesions are easier to detect in colour-coded images, but the recognition and classification of the lesion, once detected, is more easily performed on analogue images, Thus, in this difficult area of data display and image interpretation, there are perhaps no clear answers but rather a set of options with the ideal choice dependent on the problem in hand.

One important aspect of image interpretation where the physicist has already made a useful contribution, and can be expected to continue to do so, is that of data processing. The severe restrictions placed on the amount of data available in the form of recorded counts by the need to limit radiation exposure to the patient means that the most sophisticated analytical methods are sometimes required to extract the maximum amount of information. The need for new methods of data filtering and image enhancement in connection with monoclonal antibody imaging has already been mentioned.

The wide availability of reasonably priced data processing facilities has made such analyses possible. Current work may be considered under three categories. First is application to conventional images and in particular dynamic studies. There is renewed interest in functional imaging (Mac-Intyre *et al.*, 1981), and this is an area which may prove particularly interesting in the near future. Secondly, in SPECT a large amount of work· on data manipulation remains to be done. The availability of high speed digital array processors now provides facilities for successive iterations, optimisation of the iterative damping factor, attenuation correction, successive iterations coupled with attenuation correction and Fourier filtering of collected data. It is also possible to apply the technique of maximum entropy data analysis developed by Kemp (1981) and to investigate the broader and more general problems of how three-dimensional data can best be displayed in two dimensions. Finally, data analysis in positron emission tomography provides several interesting challenges such as software correction of scatter coincidence and the development of time-of-flight algorithms to improve image quality. However, such work remains more appropriate to laboratory investigations rather than routine hospital application at the present time.

Evaluation of imaging techniques in the clinical situation has received far less attention than evaluation of performance using test objects, undoubtedly because of the greatly increased complexity of the problem. Nevertheless, the ability to provide more accurate diagnostic information remains the ultimate criterion by which any innovative technique must be judged. Fortunately, this is now being recognised and an increasing number of papers are appearing in which a serious attempt has been made to assess the value of an investigation in numerical terms. A typical example is the recent work of Cinotti *et al.* (1983), who looked at the diagnostic value of image processing in myocardial scintigraphy. Data processing involved digitization, nine-point smoothing, background subtraction by linear interpolation, stationary filtering and combinations of these methods. Analysis of results showed that the stationary filter significantly increased the diagnostic value for detection of stenosis in a left anterior descending artery for a large range of disease prevalence.

Many modern approaches to data evaluation are based on receiver operator characteristic (ROC) methodology, and for a good recent view of this subject the reader is referred to Metz (1985). As a final remark on this subject, whilst the importance of proper evaluation must be emphasised, it is also important to realise that prospective trials are not necessary for really substantial medical advances—there has never been a need for a controlled clinical trial on penicillin!

In conclusion, *in vivo* imaging using small quantities of radioactive materials has been firmly established as an integral component of diagnostic medicine. Although its peak growth has now probably passed, there are a number of potentially interesting developments which should ensure that, in spite of pressure from other forms of diagnostic investigation, the importance of nuclear medicine is assured for many years.

References

Budinger, T. F. (1982). Single photon emission tomography. *In* "Nuclear Medicine and Biology" (C. Raynaud, ed.), Vol. 2, pp. 1159–1177. Pergamon Press, Oxford.

Budinger, T. F. (1983). Time of flight positron emission tomography—status relative to conventional CT. *J. Nucl. Med.* **24**, 73–77.

Cinotti, L., Meignan, N., Usdin, J. P., Vasile, N. and Castaigne, A. (1983). Diagnostic value of image processing in myocardial scintigraphy. *J. Nucl. Med.* **24**, 768–774.

Esser, P. D., ed. (1983). "Emission Computed Tomography: Current Trends". Society of Nuclear Medicine, New York.

Hill, T. C., Holman, L., Lovett, R., O'Leary, D. H., Front, D., Magistretti, P., Zimmerman, R. E., Moore, S., Clouse, M, E., Wu, J. L., Lin, T. H. and Baldwin, R. M. (1982). Initial experience with SPECT (single photon computerised emission tomography) of the brain using *N* isopropyl I-123 *p* iodoamphetamine. *J. Nucl. Med.* **23**, 191–195.

Jahangir, S. M., Brill, A. B., Bizais, Y. J. C. and Rowe, R. W. (1983). Count-rate variations with orientation of camera detector. *J. Nucl. Med.* **24**, 356–359.

Kasal, B., Sharp, P. F. and Dendy, P. P. (1983). Relationship between objective and subjective assessment of gamma camera images. *Phys. Med. Biol.* **28**, 1127–1134.

Kaye, S. B. (1981). Lipsomes—problems and promise as selective drug carriers. *Cancer Treat. Rev.* **8**, 27–50.

Kemp, M. C. (1981). Maximum entropy reconstructions in emission tomography. *In* "Medical Radionuclide Imaging 1980," Vol. 1, pp. 313–323. IAEA, Vienna.

Kirsch, C. M., Doliwa, R., Buell, U. and Roedler, D. (1983). Comparison of resting single photon emission tomography with invasive angiography. *J. Nucl. Med.* **24**, 761–767.

Kuhl, D. E., Barrior, J. R., Huang, S. C., Selin, C., Ackerman, R. F., Lear, J. L., Wu, J. L., Lin, T. H. and Phelps, M. E. (1982). Quantifying local cerebal blood flow by n-isopropyl p 123-I iodoamphetamine (IMP) tomography. *J. Nucl. Med.* **23**, 196–203.

Larson, S. M., Brown, J. P., Wright, P. W., Carrasquillo, J. A., Hellström, I, and Hellström, K. E. (1983). Imaging of melanoma with 131-I labelled monoclonal antibodies. *J. Nucl. Med.* **24**, 123–129.

MacIntyre, W. J., Cook, S. A. and Go, R. T. (1981). The future of functional imaging: Success or failure? *In* "Medical Radionuclide Imaging 1980" Vol. 1, pp. 401–417. IAEA, Vienna.

Metz, C. E. (1985) ROC curve methodology. *In* "Efficacy of Diagnostic Radiology: State of the Art Evaluation", Report of NCRP Committee #69. National Council on Radiation Protection and Measurements, Bethesda, Maryland (in press).

Mould, R. F., ed. (1983). "Quality Control of Nuclear Medicine Instrumentation". The Hospital Physicists Association, London.

Phelps, M. (1981). Positron computed tomography studies of cerebral glucose metabolism in man: theory and applications in nuclear medicine. *Semin. Nucl. Med.* **9**, 32–49.

Profitt, R. T., Williams, L. E., Presant, C. A., Tin, G. W., Uliana, J. A., Gamble, R. C. and Baldeschwieler, J. D. (1983). Tumour imaging potential of lipsomes loaded with In-111 NTA. Biodistribution in mice. *J. Nucl. Med.* **24,** 45–55.

Rougeot, H., Rozière, G. and Verat, M. (1982). Progress in image intensifier solid state localiser gamma cameras. *In* "Nuclear Medicine and Biology" (C. Raynaud, ed.), Vol. 2, pp. 1542–1545. Pergamon Press, Oxford.

Smalling, R. W. (1983). The spectrum of thallium-201 imaging in coronary artery disease. *J. Nucl. Med.* **24,** 854–856.

Smedley, H. M., Finan, P., Lennox, E. S., Ritson, A., Takei, F., Wraight, P. and Sikora, K. (1983). Localisation of metastatic carcinoma by a radiolabelled monoclonal antibody. *Br. J. Cancer* **47,** 253–259.

WHO (1982). "Quality Assurance in Nuclear Medicine". WHO, Geneva.

Zanzonico, P. B., Bigler, R. E. and Schmall, B. (1983). Neuroleptic binding—specific labelling in mice with 18-F haloperidol, a potential tracer for positron emission tomography. *J. Nucl. Med.* **24,** 408–416.

Index